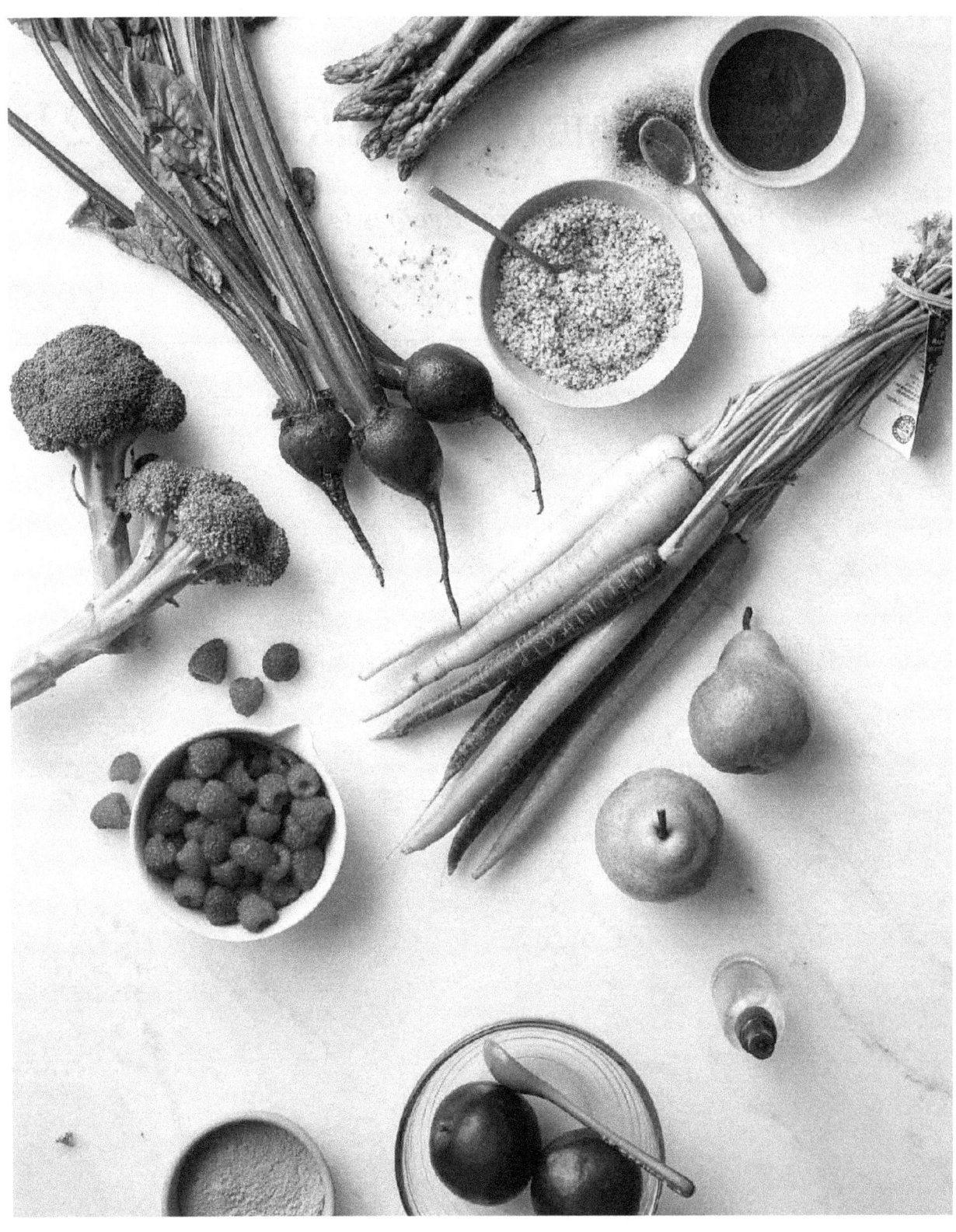

The Green Juicing Cookbook 2021

75 Energetic and Natural Recipes to Lose Weight

Copyright © 2021

No part of this publication may be reproduced, stored in a retrieval system, or transmitted in any form or by any means, electronic, mechanical, photocopying, recording, scanning, or otherwise.

Limit of Liability/Disclaimer of Warranty: The Publisher and the author make no representations or warranties with respect to the accuracy or completeness of the contents of this work and specifically disclaim all warranties, including without limitation warranties of fitness for a particular purpose. No warranty may be created or extended by sales or promotional materials. The advice and strategies contained herein may not be suitable for every situation. This work is sold with the understanding that the Publisher is not engaged in rendering medical, legal, or other professional advice or services. If professional assistance is required, the services of a competent professional person should be sought. Neither the Publisher nor the author shall be liable for damages arising herefrom. The fact that an individual, organization, or website is referred to in this work as a citation and/or potential source of further information does not mean that the author or the Publisher endorses the information the individual, organization, or website may provide or recommendations they/it may make. Further, readers should be aware that websites listed in this work may have changed or disappeared between when this work was written and when it is read.

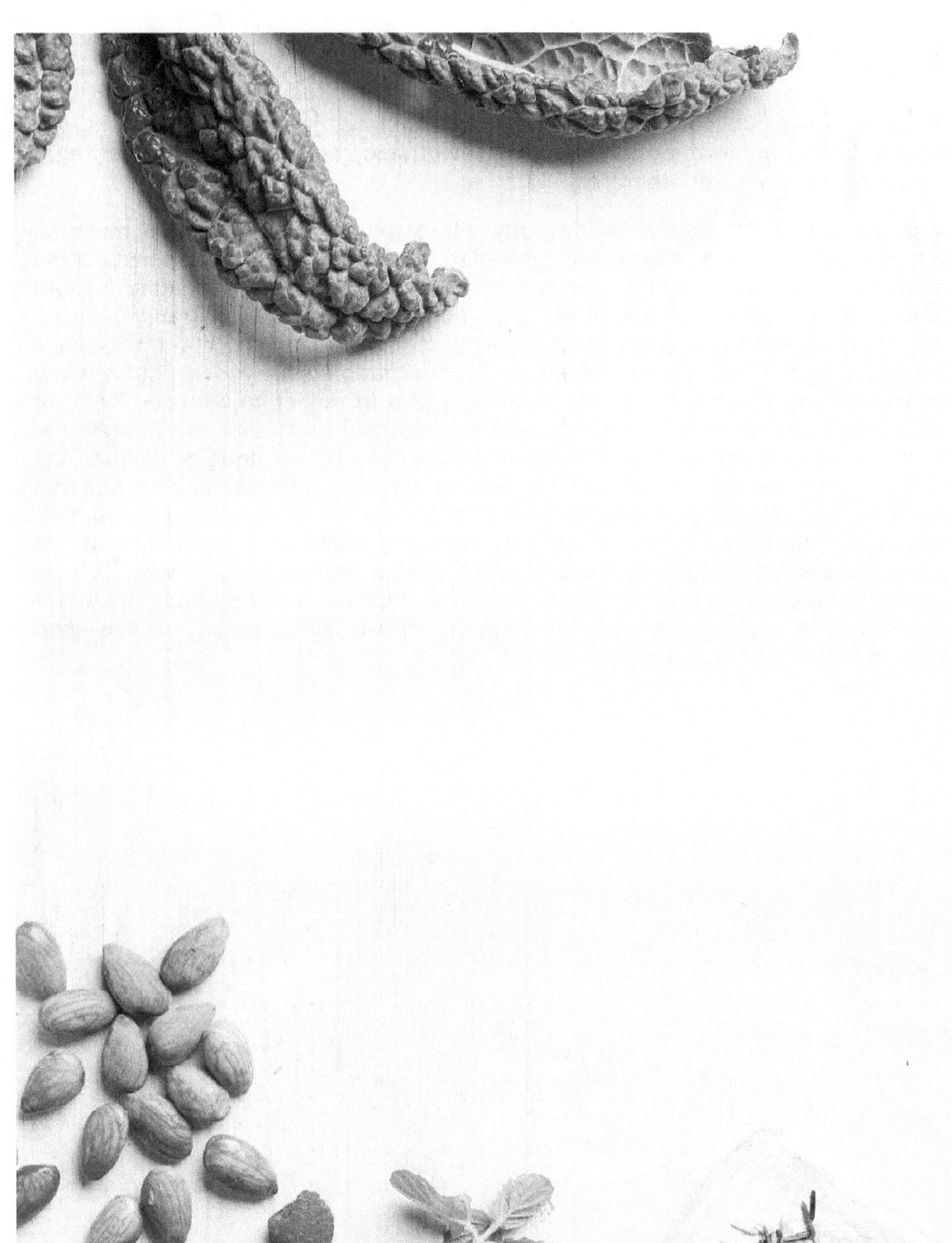

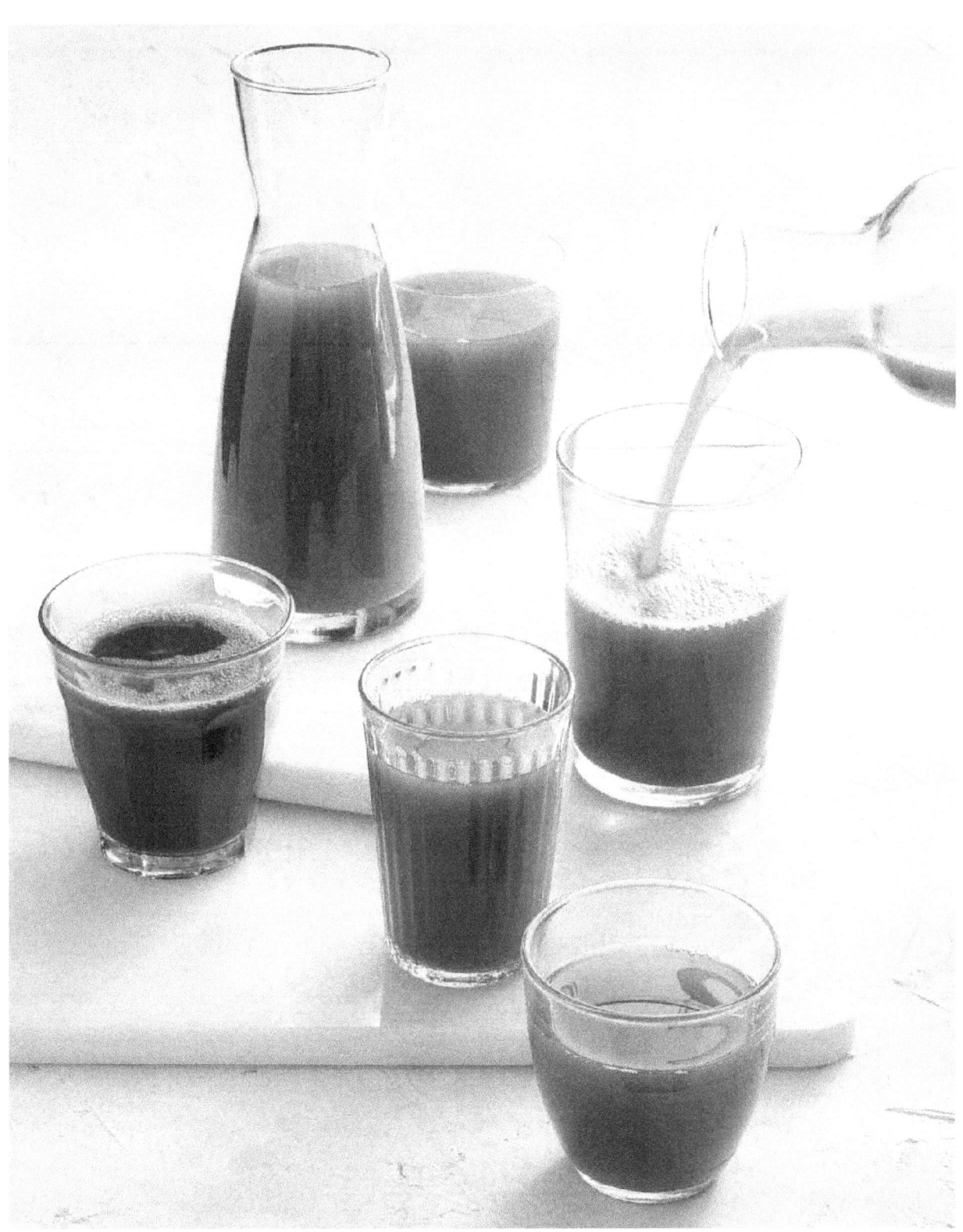

CONTENTS

INTRODUCTION

1
The Basics

2
Going Green

3
Start Your Day Green

Celery Twist Juice
Celery Refresher
Green Power
Keep It Simple Green Juice
Green Hydrating Juice
Mellow Celery
Sunrise Special
Verde Bliss
Blue Green Lemonade
Arugula Green Juice
Rejuvenator Green Juice
Tropical Island Detox Juice

4
Green Weight Loss

Slimmer Me Juice
Lean Green Juice
Mint Green Love
Bright Detox Juice
Herbal Green Juice

Matcha Green Juice
Spiced Pear Juice
Asparagus Apple Juice
Looking Good, Feeling Good
Heavenly Delight
Green Metamorphosis
Enlighten Me Juice

5
Get Skin Glowing with Green
Royal Green
Green Healing Juice
Skin Detox Juice
Happy Face Green Juice
Angelica's Green Juice
Timeless Beauty Juice
Three Cheers for Kiwi
Clear Skin Juice
Sparkling Blackberry Green Juice
Antioxidant Supreme
Grapes and Greens
Tomatillo Green Mary

6
Energize with Green
Electrolyte Power Juice
Wheatgrass Supreme
Seize the Day
Get Your Juice On
Green Extreme
Green Protein Power
Juice of Champions
Daily Endurance Juice
Peaches and Herbs Juice
Motivate Me
Make My Day Juice
Stay Rad Green Juice

7
Green Immunity
Down to Earth Juice
Ulcer Care
Anti-Inflammatory Juice
Simple Detox Juice
Greens 'n' Garlic
Cleanse Assist
Ginger Blast
Immunity Plus
Aloe Cleanser
Good, Good, Good Digestion
Vitamin C Celebration
Healthy Healing Greens

8
Your Daily Dose of Green
Beta-Carotene Greens
Alkalizing Greens
Vegetable 8
Salad in a Glass
Green Turbo
Veggies 'n' Sprouts
Kitchen Sink Green Juice
Slice of Life
Live Well Green Juice
Chlorophyll Boost
Epic Green Juice
I Dream of Green
Now and Zen Green Juice
Emerald Alkalizing Juice
The Daily Fix

9
The Three-Day Green Cleanse

THE DIRTY DOZEN™ AND THE CLEAN FIFTEEN™

MEASUREMENT CONVERSIONS

INTRODUCTION

Weight loss, glowing skin, and increased energy are just some of the wellness benefits you will get from adding green juice to your diet. The 75 recipes included in this cookbook are great and improve your well-being every day.

After squeezing the positive power of healthy vegetables, you'll wonder why you didn't start juicing earlier. Find out how to select the right juicer based on your individual needs, enhance your juices with superfoods and get all your key juice questions answered.

The green juice cookbook includes:

- Blend: Discover ways sipping different juices supports detoxification for a healthy immune system, reduces the signs of aging, and helps your skin glow.
- Vegetables and more: over 70 sample recipes from across the color spectrum using naturally sweet ingredients like oranges, blackberries and blueberries.
- Nutrition at a Glance: Make it easy to track your health with information like calories per serving, total fat, and sugar.

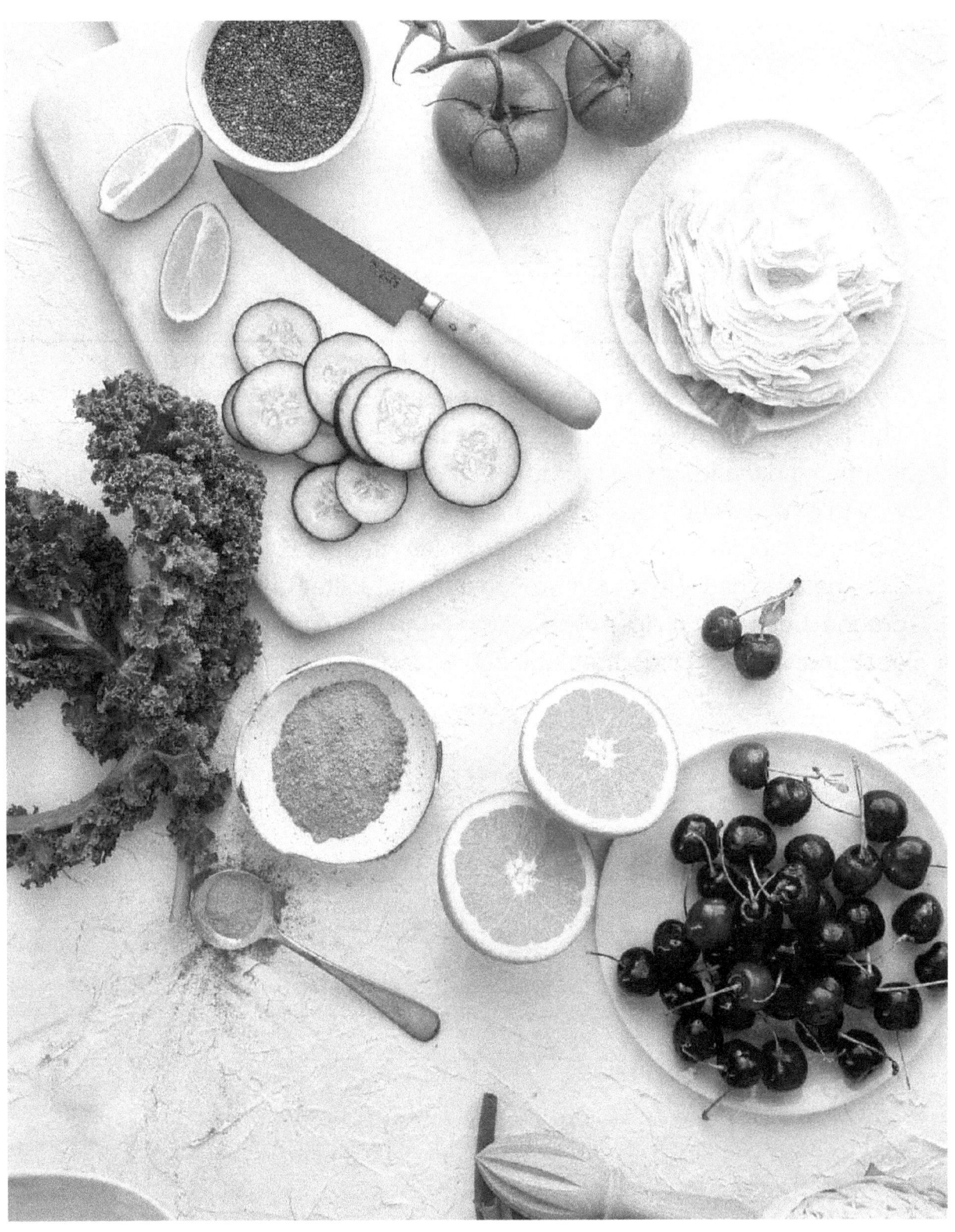

1
The Basics

Green juicing may seem like a recent health fad, but the concept of extracting nutrients from fruits and vegetables dates back to 150 BC. The first modern juicers were designed and produced in the 1930s, but in the last decade, green juicing has gained momentum as a bona fide way to get your daily dose of vitamins and minerals. Many people have reported experiencing more energy, better sleep, less stress, glowing skin, better digestion, and improved immunity after drinking their greens. Let's take a closer look at the benefits of green juicing and the best practices for incorporating it into your daily routine.

WHAT IS GREEN JUICING?

Green juice is the result of separating the liquid nutrients from the insoluble fiber of raw green vegetables. This green liquid is an excellent source of vitamins, minerals, trace elements, enzymes, and other phytonutrients that the body needs for cell regeneration and healing.

Juicing is a popular way for people to heal from health conditions that can be improved through diet. I began juicing because I wanted a natural remedy to battle my lack of energy and depression. I've met others who have reversed fibromyalgia, irritable bowel syndrome, and even eczema.

The obvious question is: Why drink vegetables instead of eating them? The answer is that our bodies need nutrients in an easily digestible form. Whole foods need to be broken down by chewing and digesting before the nutrients are available to the body. In juices, the fiber—the part of the vegetable that needs to be chewed and digested—has been removed, so the body can absorb the nutrients quickly. Some people say they can feel their green juice kicking in as soon as they drink it. Juices shouldn't completely replace whole foods, but you would have to eat a lot of vegetables to consume the amount of nutrition that's packed into just one glass of green juice.

You may have wondered what the difference is between green juicing and regular juicing. Green juices have a higher concentration of green vegetables and contain fewer fruits than other varieties of juices. Typically, a green juice is at least 75 percent vegetables (mostly leafy greens like kale and spinach) and 25 percent fruits. While many green juices appear green in color, some may take on the color of other prominent vegetables in the juice such as carrots, beets, and tomatoes. The true value of green juice is measured by the content of greens in the recipe and not the actual color of the juice.

One of the primary reasons to drink green juices instead of other juices is because green juices have a high chlorophyll content. Chlorophyll is the green pigment in plants that is responsible for converting sunlight into chemical energy to support plant growth. The molecular structure of chlorophyll resembles that of hemoglobin in human red blood cells, so chlorophyll is absorbed well by our bodies. According to an article on Dr. Josh Axe's website, chlorophyll helps detoxify the liver and heal wounds, and may even reduce the risk of cancer.

GREEN JUICES FOR HEALTH

Though your body can regenerate cells and often heal itself, it requires fuel, and fresh green juices are the purest form of nutrition for this purpose. Don't take my word for it. Ask veteran juicers, and they will cite many of the following benefits.

Green juices support gut health. Many experts believe the body's wellness can be traced to the gut. Nutrient deficiencies and toxins contribute to chronic digestive conditions, such as irritable bowel syndrome, Crohn's disease, and ulcerative colitis. Green juice, with its fortifying and detoxifying properties, corrects a gut imbalance.

Green juices give you energy. When your body has all the necessary nutrients to perform at high levels, it doesn't have to slow down and conserve energy. Green juices, stocked full of vitamins and minerals, are the perfect go-to drink for all-day energy.

Green juices support detoxification for a healthy immune system. Your body is exposed to toxins every day. Even your liver, the main organ that helps eliminate these toxins, can get overloaded. The ingredients in green juices support liver functioning and cleanse the body.

Green juices reduce the signs of aging. Antioxidants are essential to vibrant health, including glowing skin. Fruits and vegetables contain a variety of antioxidants that help fight free radicals, protect cells, hydrate the body, and reduce inflammation.

Green juices enhance weight loss. When your body is healthy, it functions at a much faster and more efficient rate. The nutrients in green juices can boost metabolism and support weight loss.

Juices vs. Smoothies

JUICES
- Can provide the nutritional equivalent of several servings of fruits and vegetables in one glass
- Lack insoluble fiber, so nutrients pass easily into the bloodstream
- Ease digestion
- Provide a quick burst of energy

SMOOTHIES
- Tend to have a high number of calories per glass
- Include lots of sugary fruits
- May contain dairy, which is problematic for some people
- Provide a slow, sustained release of nutrients

DAILY JUICING

Drinking green juice is a great way to boost a healthy diet. The US Department of Agriculture's dietary guidelines recommend that adults who consume 2,000 calories per day eat 2 cups of fruit and 2½ cups of vegetables. Green juice is meant to supplement but not replace these requirements. I like to think of green juice as a daily dose of vitamins, though the juice's nutritional value will vary depending on its ingredients.

Many people ask me if it is safe to juice every day. Absolutely! If you follow the guidelines and recipes in this book—including using no more than 25 percent fruit in the drink—one serving of juice in the morning will give you a boost of energy and mental clarity. A glass of juice in the morning also can help reduce food cravings later in the day. To get the most benefits, consume the juice first thing in the morning, include a variety of leafy green vegetables, and limit the amount of fruit. (Using too much fruit can lead to spikes in blood sugar levels.) Some experts also suggest you "chew" your juice because they believe moving your jaw stimulates the digestive process.

Be sure to check with your doctor before starting a new diet regimen, including juicing. Those who are pregnant or nursing, experiencing chronic health conditions, or have weakened immune systems should monitor their nutrition with the help of a professional.

Recommended Daily Serving for Vegetables

According to a 2017 report by the Centers for Disease Control, just 1 in 10 adults met the federal fruit or vegetable recommendations, which puts them at risk for chronic diseases such as diabetes, heart disease, some cancers, and obesity.

The US Department of Agriculture suggests the amount of vegetables you need depends on your age and gender.

CHILDREN AGE 2 TO 3: 1 cup for either gender

CHILDREN AGE 4 TO 8: 1½ cups for either gender

CHILDREN AGE 9 TO 13: 2 cups for a girl and 2½ cups for a boy

TEENS AGE 14 TO 18: 2½ cups for a girl and 3 cups for a boy

ADULTS AGE 19 TO 50: 2½ cups for a woman and 3 cups for a man

ADULTS 51 AND OLDER: 2 cups for a woman and 2½ cups for a man

The phrase "five a day" is a simple way to remember to eat your veggies. Five servings of vegetables, or 2½ cups, is easily achieved with a juice in the morning, a salad at lunch, and a cooked vegetable with dinner.

GETTING STARTED

There are many reasons to make your own green juices at home. Juices are always fresh if you make them in your kitchen and drink them right away. It's cheaper to purchase your own ingredients and make green juice in bulk rather than buy premade juice at the grocery store or local juice bar. Premade juices also contain extra sugars and preservatives to make them taste sweet, last longer, and appear brighter and more appetizing. Luckily for you, getting started is easy. You need only a few tools.

Your main tool—and investment—is a juicer, which is different from a blender because it separates the juice (nutrients) from the insoluble fiber. Later in this chapter, I'll detail different types of juicers.

You probably already have the other tools handy. A good quality knife will make prepping your produce much easier and safer. It's also a good idea to have a cutting board and a large bowl to hold all the veggies for juicing. If you intend to juice in bulk, I recommend purchasing several widemouthed glass jars with sealing lids.

Guidelines for Green Juicing

BUYING

Buy organic vegetables whenever possible to reduce your exposure to toxins.

- Check online resources, such as the Environmental Working Group's website, for shopper's guides to pesticides in produce.
- Use your senses to buy produce that looks, smells, and feels fresh.

PREPPING

Prepping vegetables before juicing ensures they are free of dirt and pesticides.

- Clean your produce with a vegetable brush and veggie wash. (To make your own wash, mix 1 cup vinegar, 4 cups distilled water, and 1 tablespoon lemon juice in a spray bottle.)
- Cut your vegetables (not fruits) and store them in baggies in the refrigerator for a few days if you won't be using them immediately.

STORING

For maximum health benefits, consume or store your juice immediately.

- To store in the refrigerator, pour juice into widemouthed glass containers. Fill to the rim and seal the jars tightly.
- Stored properly in the refrigerator, fresh juices will last one to three days, depending on the juicer and the quality of the produce.
- Green juice can be frozen for a couple of months in glass containers. When filling the containers, leave a ½-inch space to allow for expansion.
- Juice pulp can be composted, dehydrated to make crackers, or used to thicken soup.

CLEANING

It is important to clean your juicer after every use.

- Clean removable juicer parts immediately with soapy water and a brush.
- Check instructions before putting juicer parts and accessories in the dishwasher.

JUICERS

Check out the kitchen appliance section of your favorite store or website, and you'll see a seemingly endless selection of juicers. No one juicer will fit every need, but there are generally two types on the market today: centrifugal and masticating.

Centrifugal juicers: These juicers get their name from the spinning action that creates the juice. The food is put into the chute, and it is sliced by a sharp blade at the bottom of a mesh basket. As the basket spins, centrifugal force pushes the vegetables to the edges, allowing only the juice to pass through. These machines can juice most types of fruits and vegetables, though the high spinning speeds may not be ideal for some of the more delicate leafy greens.

Masticating juicers: These juicers smash and "chew" fruits and vegetables into little bits. These pieces then pass through a slowly rotating gear. The juice is essentially pressed out, so these machines are sometimes referred to as "cold press" or "slow juicers." Due to the slower speeds, it may take longer to make your juice, but masticating juicers typically yield more juice than centrifugal juicers. Masticating juicers are ideal for softer fruits and vegetables, including leafy greens.

Juicers can range in price from $50 to more than $500. Centrifugal juicers are the best option for beginners with a limited budget, but good juicers are available at all price points.

Besides price, there are some other features to consider when purchasing a juicer, and it helps to ask the following questions when comparing machines:

- How much noise does the juicer make?
- How easy is assembly and cleanup?
- What type of produce can the juicer handle?
- How much space will the machine take up?

BEST PRACTICES

Once you've decided to try juicing, you'll want to establish some best practices to ensure success. A daily health routine that is consistent and enjoyable will encourage you to continue on the path to healing and happiness.

Environment is important, and your kitchen environment can either support or hinder you. Have a look around your kitchen and consider the space. If possible, set up an area dedicated to juicing that will give you quick and easy access to your refrigerator, your juicer, and a set of clean glasses and jars. Remove any tempting junk foods and make sure your produce bins in the refrigerator are clean and ready to hold lots of fruits and veggies.

Be prepared to make juice regularly. There's nothing worse than getting excited about a glass of juice, only to realize you have no fresh fruits or vegetables available. I'm most successful in sticking to my routine when I buy a week's worth of produce in advance. I choose all my recipes for the week, make a list, and shop on Saturday. When I get home, I wash the vegetables and cut them into small pieces. Then I measure out how much I need for each recipe and place the ingredients in a sealed bag in the refrigerator. In the morning, all I have to do is prep my fruits, and I'm ready to juice.

There are a couple of reasons why it is best to drink your juice in the morning on an empty stomach. The time between your last evening meal and your first morning meal is a fasting period, meaning no food is consumed. The benefits of a fasting period include weight loss, protection against disease, improved mental agility, and lower cholesterol. When you drink juice on an empty stomach, the nutrients are absorbed into your body more easily than they would be if you had a stomach full of food. Also, when you drink your juice at the same time every day, your breakfast juice eventually becomes a healthy habit.

Common Juicing Problems and Their Solutions

THE RECIPE DOESN'T PRODUCE ENOUGH JUICE. Double the recipe, use more watery vegetables, like cucumbers and celery, or buy a masticating or slow juicer that will produce more juice.

JUICE IS TOO THICK. Thick juice contains pulp. Strain your juice or clean your juicer to ensure its proper operation.

JUICE IS TOO BITTER FROM GREENS. Add ½ lemon to the juice to counterbalance the flavor.

JUICE IS TOO SWEET. Add celery, lemon, or cucumber.

FAQS

Q: How can I speed up the juicing process?

A: Compared to making a full meal, juicing is a relatively fast process. But if you're short on time in the morning, you can prep a week's worth of vegetables in advance. You also can use a centrifugal juicer that operates at high speeds and makes juice very quickly. The more rotations per minute, the faster your juicer will produce juice.

Q: Am I missing a significant amount of fiber by juicing?

A: Insoluble fiber is removed during juicing to make the nutrients more easily available for the body to use. If you continue to eat the recommended daily amount of fruits and vegetables, your body will receive all the fiber it needs to keep your digestive system healthy.

Q: What is the average cost of getting started with green juicing?

A: Your main investment will be a juicer, which can range in price from $50 to $500. Expect to buy about a week's worth of produce at a time. The cost of produce can vary depending on where you live and what foods you buy. I find that farmers markets tend to have a nice variety of fresh, seasonal, and affordable produce. On average, a glass of green juice would cost you between $2 and $5 to make at home.

Q: Do I leave the peel on my fruits and veggies when juicing? What about the seeds?

A: Leave the peel on your veggies, but wash them first to remove dirt and pesticides. Citrus fruits should be peeled. Most seeds are fine for juicing, but I recommend removing apple seeds as they may contain a small amount of toxins. Larger pits found in cherries and peaches also should be removed to avoid damaging your juicer.

Q: How long will my green juice last?

A: The nutrients in green juices degrade as soon as they are exposed to oxygen, resulting in a loss of color, aroma, and nutritional value, so drink the juice immediately after making it or store it in an airtight container in the refrigerator. Juice produced by a centrifugal juicer can be stored for up to 24 hours. If you're using a high-quality masticating juicer, which introduces less air, you can store the juice for up to three days.

Q: Can I use a blender to make juice?

A: A blender cannot make juice because it doesn't remove fiber. However, you can choose to make a vegetable drink in your blender and strain out the fiber to make it more like a juice.

Q: What fruits and vegetables should I not juice?

A: It's not recommended to juice very soft fruits, such as bananas and avocados, because they'll clog up your machine. Most vegetables are fine for juicing except for eggplants, which are too soft. I'd also suggest avoiding leeks and winter squash, which are generally too hard to pass through a juicer.

Q: What is the best time to drink juice?

A: You can drink juice at any time during the day, but you'll get the most benefits by drinking it in the morning on an empty stomach.

Q: What should I do with the juice pulp?

A: Juice pulp is the dry, fibrous material that gets separated from liquid during the juicing process. You may discard the pulp, compost it, or save it to use in healthy recipes such as vegetable pulp crackers, veggie burgers, or soup.

Q: Does juicing have any negative side effects?

A: Juicing is a very healthy practice. If your body is not used to eating healthy foods, you may feel slightly uncomfortable at first. Symptoms might include intestinal gas or slight headaches, but these should not last long. If you experience other symptoms or persistent symptoms, you may want to consult your doctor.

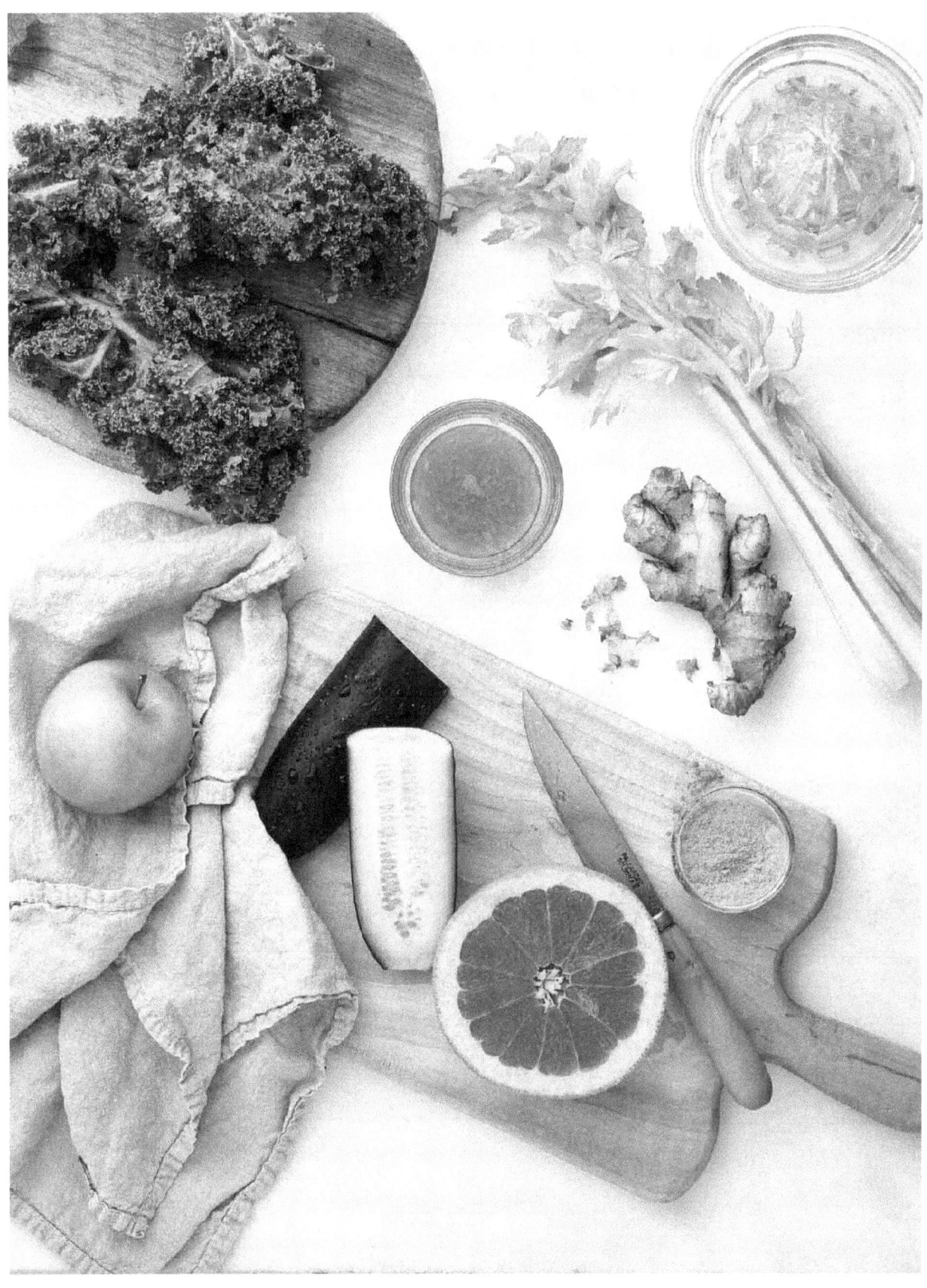

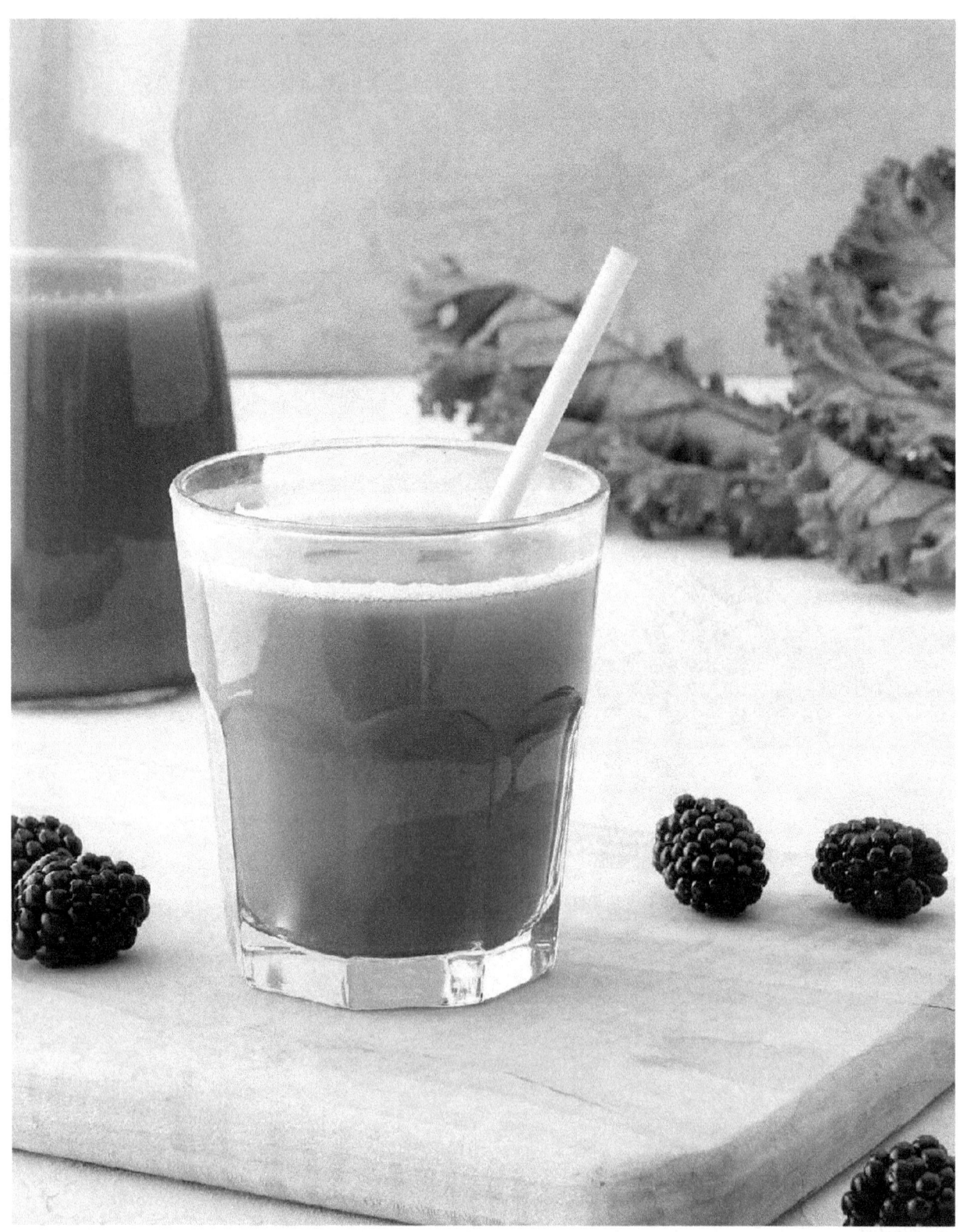

ANTIOXIDANT SUPREME

2
Going Green

When I began juicing, I had no idea how to use my juicer, and I certainly didn't know how to choose the right fruits and vegetables for my needs. I've since learned that simplicity is key, and I've arranged the information in this chapter to guide you through the juicing process. Once you know how to correctly use your juicer and understand the nutritional benefits of different fruits and vegetables, you can make recipes that will help you feel vibrant and healthy.

HOW TO MAKE A GREEN JUICE

Take some time to examine your juicer and thoroughly read its instruction manual. Practice taking the juicer apart and putting it back together to familiarize yourself with your machine.

Start with a recipe in chapter 3 of this book. Look for one with familiar ingredients that you know you like. Once you are accustomed to drinking green juice, you can try new flavors and combinations.

Buy enough produce from your local market to make juice for anyone who will be drinking it that day, keeping in mind that each recipe in this book makes a single serving.

Wash and prep your vegetables using the tips listed in "Guidelines for Green Juicing" in chapter 1. Keep in mind that the intake tubes on juicers vary. Some are small, and some are large enough to take whole apples. Make sure your fruits and veggies are cut into sizes that will fit into your juicer's intake tube.

Your juicer should come with a pitcher to collect the juice and a basket to catch the discarded pulp. If it doesn't, make sure to place a bowl or pitcher under each spout of your juicer. For easier cleanup, try placing a plastic bag inside the pulp basket.

With your pitcher in place, turn on the machine. Most juicers have one speed, but if yours has several speeds, use the lower one for softer fruits, like berries and pears, and leafy greens. Switch to higher speeds when juicing harder vegetables like carrots and beets. Be sure to juice the ingredients in the order listed in the recipe. I often like to alternate between soft and hard ingredients or put some of each into the intake tube at the same time. The harder ingredients will push the softer ones through.

What should your juice look like? A quality green juice will be rich in color, whether light green, dark green, or several colors. The juice should not be clear, though there may be some separation between nutrients and water. If the juice does separate—more likely with centrifugal juicers—stir your juice before drinking.

You might notice some foam on the surface of the juice or some bits of pulp floating around inside. The foam is the result of high-speed juicers that whip air into the juice. The foam can be spooned off the surface. If you find bits of pulp in your juice, you can still drink it, but feel free to strain the juice if this bothers you. Also check to see that your juicer is operating properly. Make sure the basket is clean and not overloaded with produce, which causes pulp to slip into your juice pitcher.

The more you make juice, the more you'll understand how your juicer functions and how to modify juices to your tastes. You might even become such a fan of juicing that, like me, you invest in several machines.

VEGETABLES AND JUICING

One of the most common myths about green juices is that they have to contain only green vegetables. While green veggies are obviously the superstars, I would be remiss if I didn't mention other vegetables that are also great for juicing. Whatever you choose, pick vegetables that produce the best taste, the most juice, and the most nutrients.

If you don't like the taste of your green juice, you're not likely to juice again. Everyone has their own preferences, so find vegetables that taste good to you. Keep in mind, though, that some veggies taste different when juiced, and you may like the taste of the juice more than the taste of the vegetable. For example, I don't like raw celery, but I love the taste of celery juice.

If you're not getting enough juice out of your vegetables, all the work put into preparing and making the juice can seem pointless, so choose at least one vegetable with a high water content. Masticating juicers also produce more juice than centrifugal juicers do.

Finally, if you're not getting much nutrition from your juice, you won't feel good about investing your time and money in this healthy habit. Thankfully, most vegetables are a great source for nutrition, so if you juice a variety of them, you'll be feeling energized and vibrant in no time.

My Top 10

Here are my top 10 vegetable picks for juicing:
- beets
- broccoli
- cabbage
- carrots
- cucumbers
- kale
- spinach
- sweet potatoes
- Swiss chard

You might be wondering if any vegetables cannot be juiced. There aren't many, but I would avoid eggplant, leeks, and winter squash for the reasons I mentioned in the FAQs in [chapter 1](). Rhubarb also could be hard on your juicer, so be sure to cut it into small pieces and test a bit of it first.

Fruit List

Here are the nutritional values and reported health benefits of commonly juiced fruits:

APPLE: vitamin C; potassium; quercetin heart health, weight loss, cancer prevention

BLACKBERRY: vitamins C and K; manganese brain health, weight loss, healthy gut, bowel regulation

BLUEBERRY: vitamins C and K; manganese; anthocyanins; quercetin heart health, brain health, blood sugar control

CHERRY: vitamin C; potassium; iron post-workout recovery, immunity boost, anti-inflammation

GRAPE: vitamins C and K; potassium cancer prevention, blood pressure regulation, chronic disease prevention

GRAPEFRUIT: vitamins C and A immunity boost, weight loss, heart health, kidney stone prevention, diabetes prevention

HONEYDEW: vitamins C, B6, and K; potassium; folate bone health, blood sugar control, skin protection, immunity boost, digestive health, blood pressure regulation

KIWI: vitamins C, K, and E; folate; potassium anti-inflammation, respiratory health, digestive health, immunity boost, eye health, blood pressure regulation

LEMON: vitamins C and B6; potassium heart health, kidney stone prevention, cancer prevention

LIME: vitamins C and B6; calcium immunity boost, kidney stone prevention, heart disease prevention

ORANGE: vitamins C and B1; folate; potassium heart health, kidney stone prevention, anemia prevention

PEACH: vitamins C, K, E, and A; potassium; niacin digestive health, heart health, skin protection, cancer prevention, allergy relief

PEAR: vitamins C and K; potassium digestive health, weight loss, immunity boost, kidney stone prevention, heart health

PINEAPPLE: vitamins C, B1, and B6; folate; copper digestive health, cancer prevention, immunity boost, anti-inflammation

PLUM: vitamins C, K, and A; potassium blood sugar control, bone health, heart health

RASPBERRY: vitamins C, K, and B; manganese; magnesium blood sugar control, weight loss, reduced joint inflammation, skin health

STRAWBERRY: vitamin C; manganese; folate heart health, blood sugar control, cancer prevention

FRUIT VS. VEGETABLES

One of the main reasons for drinking green juices is because they contain less fruit than other types of juices. But fruit isn't necessarily bad for you, and many recipes in this book contain a small amount. Experts caution that fruit juices can quickly overload your system because they contain a lot of sugar. For this reason, I recommend that your green juices have no more than 25 percent fruit. You'll eventually find that you enjoy the juice just as much without the extra sugar.

Low-sugar fruits are a perfect addition to green juice. Lemons, for instance, help balance the bitterness of sharp-tasting leafy greens. Lemons also act as a natural preservative for juices that are stored in the refrigerator. Apples and berries make great choices for green juice. These fruits contain lots of antioxidants, which promote healthy skin, protect against cancer, and encourage cell regeneration.

When you've craving a little more sweetness in your juice, try adding one green apple. The sugar content of green apples is slightly less than that of other apples, and green apples yield quite a bit of juice. As you gain juicing experience, you'll pick up little tricks like this and be able to adjust ingredients and add the right flavors to your favorite recipes.

Vegetable List

Here are the nutritional values and health benefits of commonly juiced vegetables:

ARTICHOKE: vitamins C, K, and B6; folate; magnesium; potassium cholesterol health, blood pressure regulation, liver health, digestive health

ARUGULA: vitamins C, K, and A; calcium; folate heart health, diabetes prevention, cancer prevention

ASPARAGUS: vitamins C, K, and A; folate digestive health, blood pressure regulation, weight loss

BEET: folate; manganese; potassium blood pressure regulation, heart health, digestive health, brain health

BELL PEPPER: vitamins C, K, B6, and A; potassium eye health, anemia prevention

BOK CHOY: vitamins A, C, and B6; calcium brain health, immunity boost, cancer prevention

BROCCOLI: vitamins C, B6, and A; potassium; calcium cancer prevention, cholesterol health, eye health

CABBAGE: vitamins C and K; folate; manganese anti-inflammation, digestive health, heart health, cholesterol health

CARROT: vitamins A, C, and B6; potassium eye health, skin health, cancer prevention

CAULIFLOWER: vitamins C, K, and B6; folate; potassium weight loss, bone health, cancer prevention

CELERY: vitamins K, C, and A; folate; potassium digestive health, anti-inflammation, cholesterol health, blood pressure regulation, skin health

COLLARD GREENS: vitamins A, C, K, and B6; calcium; iron cancer prevention, detox support, anti-inflammation, heart health

CUCUMBER: vitamins K and C; magnesium; potassium hydration, weight loss, blood sugar control, bowel regulation

DAIKON RADISH: vitamins C and B6; potassium digestive health, respiratory health, immunity boost, cancer prevention

DANDELION GREENS: vitamins A, C, K, and E; folate; iron; calcium anti-inflammation, detox support, blood sugar control, liver health, cancer prevention

ENDIVE: vitamins A and C; potassium digestive health, cholesterol health, bone health

FENNEL: vitamin C; potassium; manganese weight loss, heart health, cancer prevention

GREEN BEANS: vitamins C, A, and K; calcium; potassium;

phosphorus heart health, cancer prevention, diabetes prevention, bone health

KALE: vitamins A, K, and C; manganese cholesterol health, cancer prevention, eye health, weight loss

KOHLRABI: vitamin A; potassium digestive health, weight loss, anemia prevention, bone health

LETTUCE (green leaf, red leaf, romaine): vitamins A and K; potassium; zinc; folate anti-inflammation, sleep aid, anti-anxiety relief

MUSTARD GREENS: vitamins K, A, and C; calcium; potassium bone health, digestive health, detox support

OKRA: vitamins C, A, and B6; magnesium cancer prevention, heart health, diabetes prevention, digestive health

PARSNIP: vitamins C, K, and E; folate; magnesium weight loss, immunity boost

PEAS: vitamins A, K, and C; thiamine; folate blood sugar control, digestive health, heart disease prevention

POTATO: vitamins C and B6; potassium; folate heart health, digestive health, blood sugar control

PUMPKIN: vitamins A and C; potassium; copper; magnesium chronic disease prevention, immunity boost, eye health

RADISH: vitamin B6; riboflavin; calcium; folate immunity boost, digestive health, urinary tract health

RAPINI: vitamins A, C, and B6; potassium cancer prevention, bone health, heart disease prevention, detox support

RUTABAGA: vitamins C and B6; magnesium; calcium cancer prevention, anti-aging support, digestive health

SPINACH: vitamins K, A, B2, and B6; folate; manganese eye health, brain health, muscle health

SQUASH: vitamins A, C, E, and B6; niacin diabetes

management, anti-inflammation, lung health

SWEET POTATO: vitamins A and B6; magnesium; potassium digestive health, immunity boost, lung health

SWISS CHARD: vitamins A and C; magnesium cancer prevention, blood pressure regulation, bone health, brain health

TOMATO: vitamins C and K1; folate; potassium heart health, cancer prevention, skin health

TURNIP GREENS: vitamins A, C, and B6 heart health, bone health, eye health, brain health

ZUCCHINI: vitamins A, C, and K; manganese; potassium digestive health, blood sugar control, heart health, eye health

ROTATING YOUR GREENS

I talk a lot about leafy greens because they are loaded with phytonutrients and vitamins and minerals that boost your health. Greens also contain small amounts of alkaloids and phytotoxins like oxalates and goitrogens, which are naturally occurring chemicals that can build up in your body and impact your thyroid and kidney health. Don't be alarmed by this. You can get a proper balance of nutrition and avoid this risk by rotating your greens.

Green vegetables are classified according to which part of the plant is edible. The most commonly juiced green vegetables fall into these four families:

Cruciferous: These greens include favorites such as broccoli, kale, and cabbage.

Amaranth: Popular greens in this family are beetroot, spinach, and Swiss chard.

Asteraceae: Lettuces, dandelions, and artichokes belong to this family of mostly herbaceous plants.

Apiaceae: Celery, fennel, parsley, and cilantro make up the sweet herbs of this family.

Rotate your greens weekly to ensure you receive adequate nutrition. I suggest you first experiment with a few greens in each family to find out which ones you like best. Then you can try recipes using different greens, mixing and matching them to come up with your own variations of healthy and satisfying juices.

The Green List

Green vegetables get their color from chlorophyll, a pigment that is essential to plants' ability to absorb energy from sunlight. In the human body, chlorophyll has important health benefits and detoxifies the liver. Many green vegetables contain vitamins A, C, and K, as well as folate, iron, and calcium. Here are some common green vegetables, including leafy greens.

CRUCIFEROUS FAMILY

- bok choy
- broccoli
- Brussels sprouts
- cabbage
- Chinese cabbage
- collard greens
- garden cress
- horseradish greens
- kale
- kohlrabi
- mustard greens
- radish greens
- rutabaga greens
- turnip greens
- watercress

AMARANTH FAMILY

- beetroot greens
- lamb's-quarter
- spinach
- Swiss chard

ASTERACEAE FAMILY

- artichokes
- dandelions
- endive
- lettuces

APIACEAE FAMILY

- carrot greens
- celery
- cilantro
- dill
- fennel
- parsley

CUCURBIT FAMILY

- cucumber
- zucchini/courgette

LEGUME FAMILY

- alfalfa
- clover
- green beans
- peas

ENHANCE WITH SUPERFOODS

Superfoods add a powerful boost of nutrition without adding many calories. When incorporated into a well-balanced diet, these nutrient-dense ingredients offer disease-fighting and health-enhancing properties that go beyond basic nutrition. Superfoods are valued for their ability to help regulate your metabolism, reduce inflammation, and protect your organs from toxins.

Typically, superfoods are not eaten by themselves but are found in powder or liquid form, which you can add to your food or drink. The following superfoods, most of which can be found in your local supermarket, are my top juicing picks because of their exceptional nutritional value.

Aloe vera: The juice from this succulent plant contains saponins, which are natural compounds that help detoxify the body, decrease inflammation, and improve immunity.

Chia seeds: These tiny seeds are rich in omega-3 fatty acids, antioxidants, and fiber.

Chlorella: This green alga helps improve cholesterol levels and removes toxins from the body.

Flax seeds: Flax is another small seed that is packed with nutrition. These seeds are high in fiber, omega-3 fatty acids, and lignans, which may reduce your risk of cancer.

Goji berries: The powdered form of these berries is an excellent source of antioxidants with anti-aging benefits.

Hemp seeds: Consider hemp seeds, which contain all nine essential amino acids, as a valuable protein source to add to your juices.

Maca: This root, a relative of the radish, has been used for centuries to increase energy and enhance mood.

Matcha: This powdered form of green tea leaves will boost your metabolism and detoxify your body, improving immunity.

Raw cacao: Cacao has anti-inflammatory properties, promotes heart health, and may help boost your mood.

Spirulina: This type of blue-green algae is high in protein and may improve gut health.

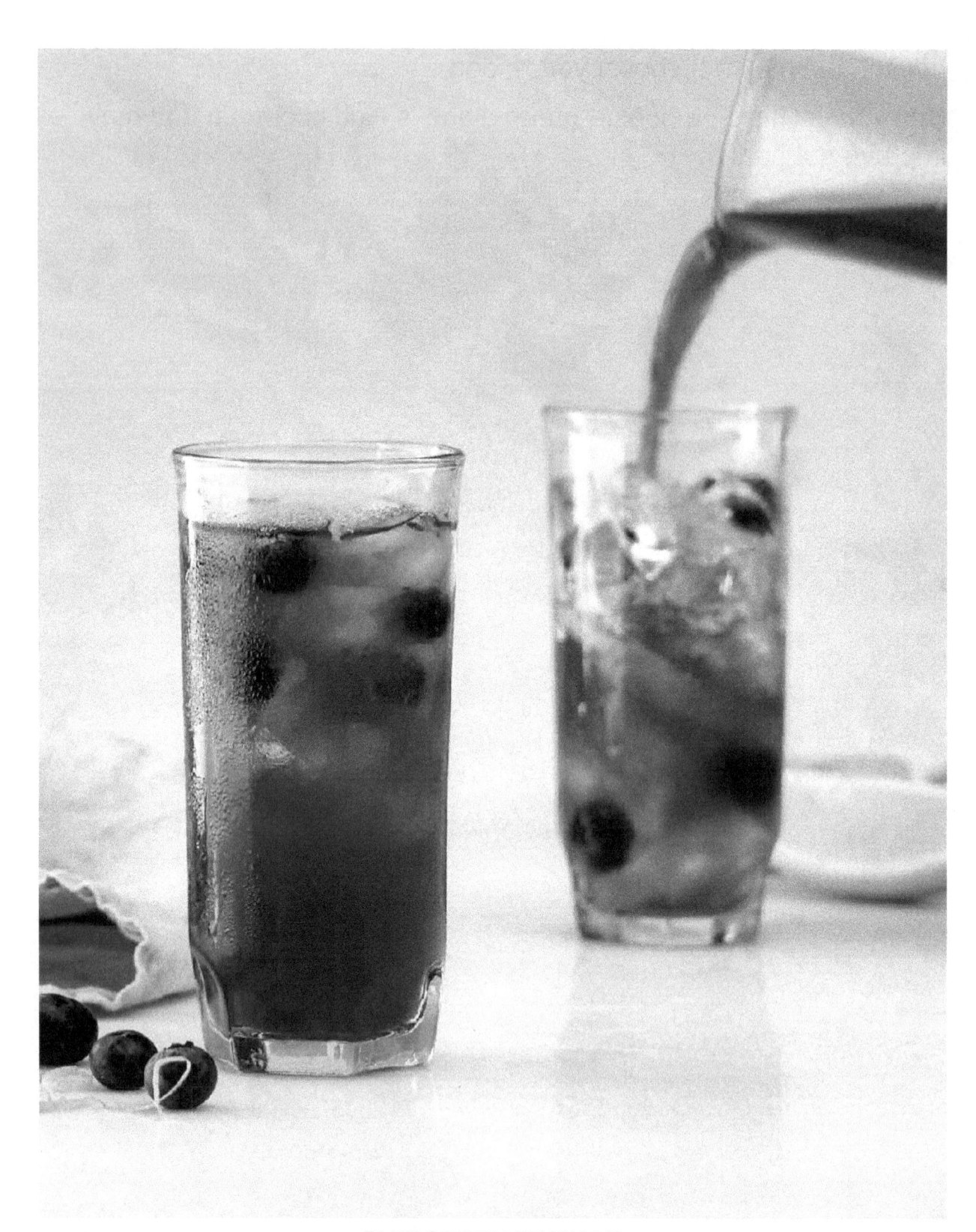

BLUE GREEN LEMONADE

3
Start Your Day Green

Celery Twist Juice

Celery Refresher

Green Power

Keep It Simple Green Juice

Green Hydrating Juice

Mellow Celery

Sunrise Special

Verde Bliss

Blue Green Lemonade

Arugula Green Juice

Rejuvenator Green Juice

Tropical Island Detox Juice

Mornings carry a certain energy of hope and possibilities. We have an opportunity to start fresh and make decisions that benefit our minds and bodies. Mornings also can bring challenges, and many of us don't have the time to devote to a complicated health routine. That's why I like to begin each day by drinking a green juice. I can make my green juice the night before so it's ready to go, giving me a quick burst of energy and nutrition in the morning when I need it most. The recipes in this chapter offer a simple and satisfying way for you to start your day.

CELERY TWIST JUICE

Makes 1 (16-ounce) serving **Prep time:** 10 minutes

Celery juice has become popular recently due to its ability to help your body heal from many types of ailments, including liver toxicity and eczema. According to best-selling author Anthony William, also known as the "Medical Medium," sodium cluster salts in celery differ from other types of sodium and can help fight off unwanted bacteria and viruses.

---

1 large bunch celery
2 clementine oranges

1. Wash all the ingredients.
2. Trim ends from the celery, then cut into 4-inch pieces.
3. Peel the clementines and separate into quarters.
4. Place a pitcher under the juicer's spout to collect the juice.
5. Feed the celery, then the clementines through the juicer's intake tube.
6. When the juice stops flowing, remove the pitcher and stir the juice.
7. Serve immediately.

INGREDIENT TIP: For best results, drink celery juice on an empty stomach. If you are not used to drinking any green juice at all, begin with 4 to 8 ounces per day.

PER SERVING: CALORIES: 96; TOTAL FAT: 1G; SUGAR: 16G; CARBOHYDRATES: 28G; FIBER: 2G; PROTEIN: 5G

CELERY REFRESHER

Makes 1 (16-ounce) serving **Prep time:** 10 minutes

Each ingredient in this refreshing juice is bursting with water and nutrients that help keep your body hydrated. Celery adds a saltiness, and citrus rounds out the juice with a sweet but tart flavor.

---

4 celery ribs
2 cucumbers
1 orange
1 lemon

1. Wash all the ingredients.
2. Trim the ends from the celery and cucumbers, then cut into 4-inch pieces.
3. Peel the orange and lemon, then cut into quarters.
4. Place a pitcher under the juicer's spout to collect the juice.
5. Feed each ingredient through the juicer's intake tube in the order listed.
6. When the juice stops flowing, remove the pitcher and stir the juice.
7. Serve immediately.

INGREDIENT TIP: Peel citrus fruits before juicing. The peel contains oils that may taste bitter and cause indigestion. The peels of conventionally grown citrus also may contain harmful pesticides.

PER SERVING: CALORIES: 141; TOTAL FAT: 1G; SUGAR: 24G; CARBOHYDRATES: 47G; FIBER: 2G; PROTEIN: 6G

GREEN POWER

Makes 1 (12-ounce) serving **Prep time:** 10 minutes

This green juice may not appear a true green color because of the carrots, but it is chock-full of antioxidants and other nutrients that benefit your eyes, brain, muscles, hair, and nails. Now that's powerful!

---

2 cups spinach
6 kale leaves
1 green apple
3 carrots
Fresh ginger root

1. Wash all the ingredients.
2. Remove the apple core and discard. Cut the apple into quarters, leaving the peel intact.
3. Cut the carrots into 4-inch pieces.
4. Slice off a ½-inch piece of the ginger root.
5. Place a pitcher under the juicer's spout to collect the juice.
6. Feed each ingredient through the juicer's intake tube in the order listed.
7. When the juice stops flowing, remove the pitcher and stir the juice.
8. Serve immediately.

STORING TIP: Carrot juice does not keep well in the refrigerator, and the color and flavor can spoil quickly. Always drink carrot juice immediately.

PER SERVING: CALORIES: 158; TOTAL FAT: 2G; SUGAR: 22G; CARBOHYDRATES: 45G; FIBER: 2G; PROTEIN: 9G

KEEP IT SIMPLE GREEN JUICE

Makes 1 (10-ounce) serving **Prep time:** 10 minutes

This is one of my favorite recipes because it uses only three ingredients and the flavors complement each other so well. Plus, I usually have these items in my refrigerator, which saves me a trip to the market.

4 romaine lettuce leaves
4 celery ribs
1 green apple

1. Wash all the ingredients.
2. Trim the ends from the celery, then and cut into 4-inch pieces.
3. Remove the apple core and discard. Cut the apple into quarters, leaving the peel intact.
4. Place a pitcher under the juicer's spout to collect the juice.
5. Feed each ingredient through the juicer's intake tube in the order listed.
6. When the juice stops flowing, remove the pitcher and stir the juice.
7. Serve immediately.

INGREDIENT TIP: You may use any variety of apple for the recipes in this book. I recommend using green apples because they contain slightly less sugar than other types of apples.

PER SERVING: CALORIES: 73; TOTAL FAT: 1G; SUGAR: 15G; CARBOHYDRATES: 23G; FIBER: 1G; PROTEIN: 2G

GREEN HYDRATING JUICE

Makes 1 (12-ounce) serving **Prep time:** 15 minutes

This is the perfect green juice if you have a demanding work schedule. Take it with you to the office and sip while you work. This juice will keep your body hydrated and your mind clear.

1 cup spinach
4 celery ribs
1 green apple
1 cucumber
½ lemon

1. Wash all the ingredients.
2. Trim the ends from the celery and cucumber, then cut into 4-inch pieces.
3. Remove the apple core and discard. Cut the apple into quarters, leaving the peel intact.
4. Peel the lemon and cut into quarters.
5. Place a pitcher under the juicer's spout to collect the juice.
6. Feed each ingredient through the juicer's intake tube in the order listed.
7. When the juice stops flowing, remove the pitcher and stir the juice.
8. Serve immediately.

VARIATION TIP: You can make this your go-to green juice by regularly swapping out your greens to get all the nutrients you need. Instead of spinach, try kale, romaine, Swiss chard, or collard greens.

PER SERVING: CALORIES: 102; TOTAL FAT: 1G; SUGAR: 19G; CARBOHYDRATES: 32G; FIBER: 1G; PROTEIN: 3G

MELLOW CELERY

Makes 1 (12-ounce) serving **Prep time:** 10 minutes

Broccoli deserves an award for its supporting role in this juice. This vegetable has a surprisingly mellow flavor, yet it has powerful effects. Broccoli helps reduce inflammation, control blood sugar, and protect against cancer.

4 celery ribs
1 cucumber
2 cups broccoli
½ lemon

1. Wash all the ingredients.
2. Trim the ends from the celery and cucumber, then cut into 4-inch pieces.
3. Remove the stalk from the broccoli crown with a knife and discard or save to juice later. Cut the crown into small florets.
4. Peel the lemon and cut into quarters.
5. Place a pitcher under the juicer's spout to collect the juice.
6. Feed each ingredient through the juicer's intake tube in the order listed.
7. When the juice stops flowing, remove the pitcher and stir the juice.
8. Serve immediately.

INGREDIENT TIP: Remove celery leaves before juicing as they may make your juice bitter.

PER SERVING: CALORIES: 148; TOTAL FAT: 2G; SUGAR: 13G; CARBOHYDRATES: 41G; FIBER: 2G; PROTEIN: 14G

SUNRISE SPECIAL

Makes 1 (10-ounce) serving **Prep time:** 10 minutes

All the ingredients in this juice will nourish the liver, which helps your body digest food and filter toxins. Drink this juice once or twice a week to keep everything running smoothly. The taste is sweet with a slight peppery kick from the parsley.

---

2 cups romaine lettuce (about 4 leaves)
2 tablespoons parsley leaves
½ green apple
½ beet
1 lemon

1. Wash all the ingredients.
2. Remove the apple core and discard. Cut the apple into quarters, leaving the peel intact.
3. Remove any greens from the beet and save for juicing later. Cut the beet into quarters.
4. Peel the lemon and cut into quarters.
5. Place a pitcher under the juicer's spout to collect the juice.
6. Feed each ingredient through the juicer's intake tube in the order listed.
7. When the juice stops flowing, remove the pitcher and stir the juice.
8. Serve immediately.

INGREDIENT TIP: Beet juice can stain your fingers and clothes. Prep and cut all your other fruits and vegetables first so you only have to clean up once.

PER SERVING: CALORIES: 63; TOTAL FAT: 1G; SUGAR: 12G; CARBOHYDRATES: 21G; FIBER: 1G; PROTEIN: 3G

VERDE BLISS

Makes 1 (10-ounce) serving **Prep time:** 15 minutes

The first time I made this juice, I was astounded by the dense green color from the spinach. Kids especially will love the color and minty aroma. The chia seeds expand and thicken the juice, giving it a distinct flavor and texture.

---

3 cups spinach
10 mint leaves
1 green apple
1 teaspoon chia seeds

1. Wash all the spinach, mint leaves, and apple.
2. Remove the apple core and discard. Cut the apple into quarters, leaving the peel intact.
3. Place a pitcher under the juicer's spout to collect the juice.
4. Feed the first three ingredients through the juicer's intake tube in the order listed.
5. When the juice stops flowing, remove the pitcher, add the chia seeds, stir the juice, and let sit for five minutes.
6. Serve immediately.

INGREDIENT TIP: You may notice your juicer doesn't produce much juice from spinach and other leafy greens. Try rolling the leaves into a ball before putting them through the intake tube.

PER SERVING: CALORIES: 74; TOTAL FAT: 1G; SUGAR: 13G; CARBOHYDRATES: 21G; FIBER: 1G; PROTEIN: 3G

BLUE GREEN LEMONADE

Makes 1 (12-ounce) serving **Prep time:** 10 minutes

This is a great recipe for introducing children and young people to green juice. The juice's color is interesting, and kids will appreciate the juice's fruity flavor without even realizing it's good for them. This drink is full of antioxidants and great for the immune system. You'll like it, too!

---

4 kale leaves
1 cucumber
1 pear
½ cup blueberries
1 lemon

1. Wash all the ingredients.
2. Trim the ends from the cucumber, then cut into 4-inch pieces.
3. Cut the pear into quarters, removing the seeds but leaving the peel intact.
4. Peel the lemon and cut into quarters.
5. Place a pitcher under the juicer's spout to collect the juice.
6. Feed each ingredient through the juicer's intake tube in the order listed.
7. When the juice stops flowing, remove the pitcher and stir the juice.
8. Serve immediately.

DID YOU KNOW? There are two common types of kale: curly and lacinato. The lacinato, or Italian, variety of kale is often called dinosaur kale because it has dark, bumpy leaves that resemble dinosaur skin.

PER SERVING: CALORIES: 187; TOTAL FAT: 2G; SUGAR: 30G; CARBOHYDRATES: 61G; FIBER: 2G; PROTEIN: 8G

ARUGULA GREEN JUICE

Makes 1 (12-ounce) serving **Prep time:** 15 minutes

If you've ever eaten a mixed salad with romaine lettuce, arugula, and pears, then you have some idea of how this juice tastes. Arugula adds a slight peppery flavor and helps lower the risk of diabetes, heart disease, and cancer.

1 romaine lettuce heart
½ cup arugula
2 pears
½ lemon

1. Wash all the ingredients.
2. Cut the pears into quarters, removing the seeds but leaving the peel intact.
3. Peel the lemon and cut into quarters.
4. Place a pitcher under the juicer's spout to collect the juice.
5. Feed each ingredient through the juicer's intake tube in the order listed.
6. When the juice stops flowing, remove the pitcher and stir the juice.
7. Serve immediately.

INGREDIENT TIP: The center of a head of romaine lettuce is called its heart. You often can find romaine hearts prewashed and packaged in groups of 2 or 3 at the grocery store.

PER SERVING: CALORIES: 181; TOTAL FAT: 1G; SUGAR: 35G; CARBOHYDRATES: 63G; FIBER: 2G; PROTEIN: 5G

REJUVENATOR GREEN JUICE

Makes 1 (12-ounce) serving **Prep time:** 15 minutes

This juice is called the rejuvenator because it's so healthy and energizing. The pink grapefruit adds a wonderful color to the juice, and the fruit is great for your heart and your skin.

½ pink grapefruit
4 kale leaves
1 cucumber
½ green apple
Fresh ginger root

1. Wash all the ingredients.
2. Peel the grapefruit and separate into sections.
3. Trim the ends from the cucumber, then cut into 4-inch pieces.
4. Remove the apple core and discard. Cut the apple into quarters, leaving the peel intact.
5. Slice off a 1-inch piece of the ginger root.
6. Place a pitcher under the juicer's spout to collect the juice.
7. Feed each ingredient through the juicer's intake tube in the order listed.
8. When the juice stops flowing, remove the pitcher and stir the juice.
9. Serve immediately.

HEALTH TIP: Be sure to check with your doctor before consuming grapefruit, which can interact with certain medications.

PER SERVING: CALORIES: 121; TOTAL FAT: 1G; SUGAR: 17G; CARBOHYDRATES: 33G; FIBER: 1G; PROTEIN: 6G

TROPICAL ISLAND DETOX JUICE

Makes 1 (12-ounce) serving **Prep time:** 10 minutes

Drinking this juice is like enjoying a fruity drink on a tropical island. The added benefit is that you'll hydrate and detox your body with the green power of kale and chlorella.

---

2 oranges
8 kale leaves
1 teaspoon chlorella powder
4 ounces coconut water

1. Wash the oranges and kale leaves.
2. Peel the oranges and cut into quarters.
3. Place a pitcher under the juicer's spout to collect the juice.
4. Feed the oranges, then the kale through the juicer's intake tube.
5. When the juice stops flowing, remove the pitcher, add the chlorella powder and coconut water, and stir the juice.
6. Serve immediately.

INGREDIENT TIP: Chlorella can be purchased at a health food store or online. Be sure to buy brands without fillers or preservatives, which may contaminate this superfood.

PER SERVING: CALORIES: 151; TOTAL FAT: 2G; SUGAR: 23G; CARBOHYDRATES: 41G; FIBER: 2G; PROTEIN: 11G

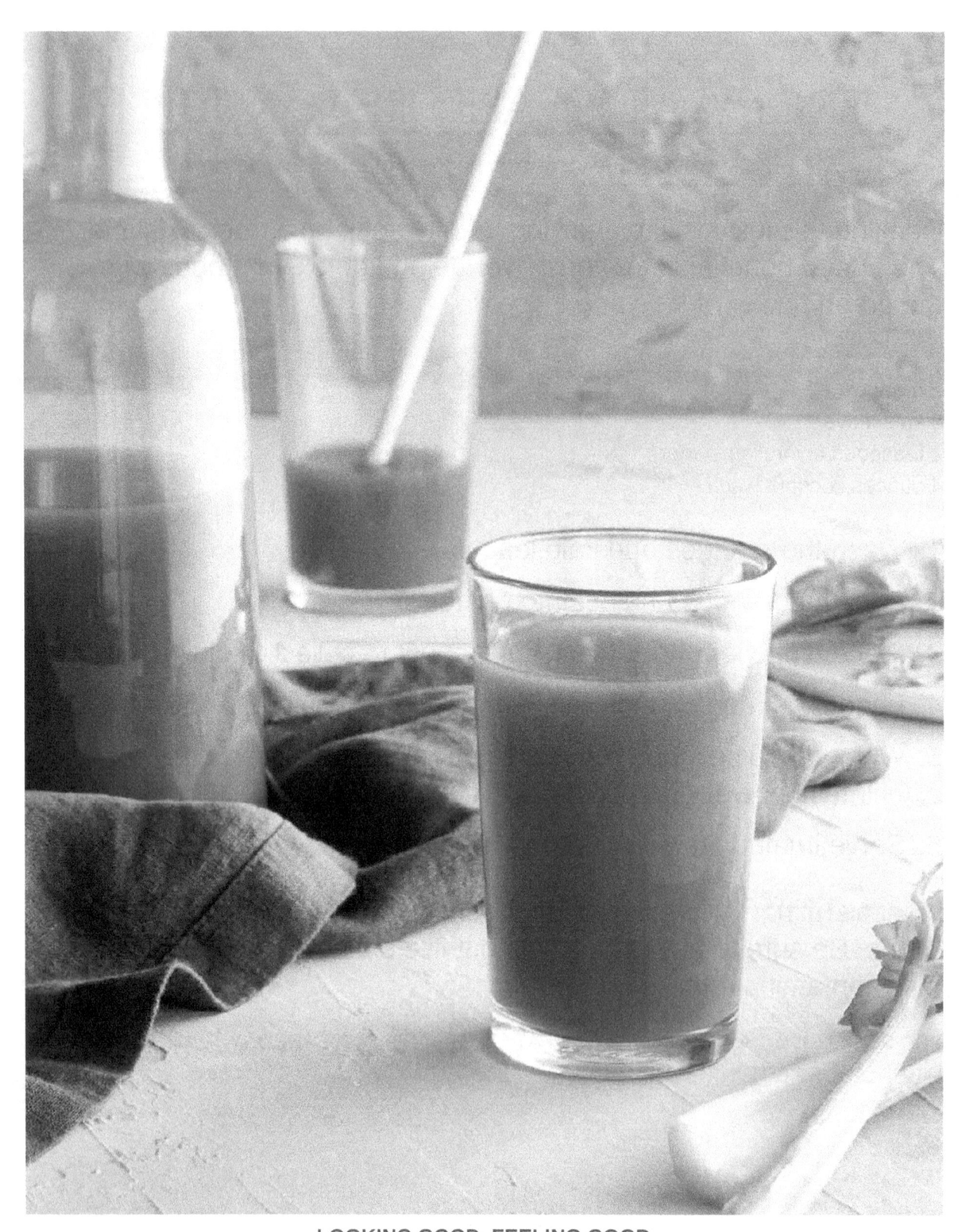

LOOKING GOOD, FEELING GOOD

4
Green Weight Loss

Slimmer Me Juice

Lean Green Juice

Mint Green Love

Bright Detox Juice

Herbal Green Juice

Matcha Green Juice

Spiced Pear Juice

Asparagus Apple Juice

Looking Good, Feeling Good

Heavenly Delight

Green Metamorphosis

Enlighten Me Juice

All the green juice recipes in this book promote healthy weight. A single green juice contains few calories and lots of nutrients. When your body is nourished with the vitamins and minerals it needs to thrive, you are less likely to crave sweets and junk food. Instead, you will feel energetic, alert, and optimistic. The recipes in this chapter target these goals so you can progress quickly and stay motivated to reach your ideal weight.

SLIMMER ME JUICE

Makes 1 (12-ounce) serving **Prep time:** 15 minutes

Honeydew melons contain few calories. They also burst with flavor and have a high water content, making them an ideal food for weight loss. This sweet juice is high in potassium and vitamins A, B, C, and K.

2 cups mixed greens
¼ honeydew
melon 1 cucumber
1 lemon

1. Wash all the ingredients.
2. Cut the honeydew melon in half. Scoop out seeds with a spoon. Remove the rind and discard. Cut the melon into quarters.
3. Trim the ends from the cucumber, then cut into 4-inch pieces.
4. Peel the lemon and cut into quarters.
5. Place a pitcher under the juicer's spout to collect the juice.
6. Feed each ingredient through the juicer's intake tube in the order listed.
7. When the juice stops flowing, remove the pitcher and stir the juice.
8. Serve immediately.

HEALTH TIP: Proper hydration is important for maintaining a strong body and healthy weight. Make sure you drink at least 8 glasses of water per day in addition to your daily green juice.

PER SERVING: CALORIES: 113; TOTAL FAT: 1G; SUGAR: 23G; CARBOHYDRATES: 33G; FIBER: 1G; PROTEIN: 4G

LEAN GREEN JUICE

Makes 1 (12-ounce) serving **Prep time:** 15 minutes

A healthy digestive tract is key to maintaining overall health and a healthy weight. Apples boost good gut bacteria and contain pectin, a soluble fiber that improves digestion. Collard greens contain antioxidants that protect the stomach lining, and fennel soothes the digestive process. Stay lean with green juice.

---

1 green apple
5 collard leaves
1 cucumber ¼
fennel bulb 2
celery ribs ½
lemon Fresh
ginger root

1. Wash all the ingredients.
2. Remove the apple core and discard. Cut the apple into quarters, leaving the peel intact.
3. Trim the ends from the cucumber and celery, then cut into 4-inch pieces.
4. Remove the stalks and fronds from the fennel and save for later. Cut the bulb into quarters.
5. Peel the lemon and cut into quarters.
6. Slice off a ½-inch piece of the ginger root.
7. Place a pitcher under the juicer's spout to collect the juice.
8. Feed each ingredient through the juicer's intake tube in the order listed.
9. When the juice stops flowing, remove the pitcher and stir the juice.
10. Serve immediately.

INGREDIENT TIP: All the parts of fennel are edible. The bulb, leaves, and stems can be juiced and the seeds can be used to flavor meats, vegetables, salads, and baked goods.

PER SERVING: CALORIES: 106; TOTAL FAT: 1G; SUGAR: 17G; CARBOHYDRATES: 33G; FIBER: 1G; PROTEIN: 4G

MINT GREEN LOVE

Makes 1 (10-ounce) serving **Prep time:** 15 minutes

Mint green is the color and the flavor of this aromatic and healthy juice. The pineapple and the coconut water contain enzymes that aid digestion and boost metabolism, making this juice a must-have for anyone who wants to lose weight.

---

1 cup pineapple
4 large lettuce leaves
15 mint leaves
½ cup coconut water

1. Wash the lettuce and mint.
2. Trim the ends and skin from the pineapple, then remove the core and discard. Cut pineapple into 1-inch chunks.
3. Place a pitcher under the juicer's spout to collect the juice.
4. Feed the first three ingredients through the juicer's intake tube in the order listed.
5. When the juice stops flowing, remove the pitcher, add the coconut water, and stir.
6. Serve immediately.

INGREDIENT TIP: Freeze your coconut water in ice cube trays to use later in water, juice, or tea.

PER SERVING: CALORIES: 71; TOTAL FAT: 1G; SUGAR: 14G; CARBOHYDRATES: 21G; FIBER: 1G; PROTEIN: 2G

BRIGHT DETOX JUICE

Makes 1 (12-ounce) serving **Prep time:** 15 minutes

Pineapple is bright and tastes fresh. It also contains the enzyme bromelain, which relieves inflammation and helps with poor digestion. Choose this juice for a dynamic weight loss and detoxification combo.

---

1 cup pineapple
1 cup spinach
1 cup chopped lettuce leaves
1 cucumber
10 sprigs cilantro

1. Wash all the ingredients except the pineapple.
2. Trim the ends and skin from the pineapple, then remove the core and discard. Cut pineapple into 1-inch chunks.
3. Trim the ends from the cucumber, then cut into 4-inch pieces.
4. Place a pitcher under the juicer's spout to collect the juice.
5. Feed each ingredient through the juicer's intake tube in the order listed.
6. When the juice stops flowing, remove the pitcher and stir the juice.
7. Serve immediately.

DID YOU KNOW? Not all lettuces have the same nutritional value. For instance, one cup of romaine lettuce contains 23 percent of the daily vitamin A requirement, but iceberg lettuce contains only 2 percent.

PER SERVING: CALORIES: 87; TOTAL FAT: 1G; SUGAR: 15G; CARBOHYDRATES: 25G; FIBER: 1G; PROTEIN: 3G

HERBAL GREEN JUICE

Makes 1 (12-ounce) serving **Prep time:** 20 minutes

Believe it or not, dandelions are herbs and detoxifying ones at that. They taste like most other greens, earthy and slightly bitter, but the orange and green tea in this juice round out the flavor for a smooth finish.

¾ cup green tea, cooled
10 dandelion greens
10 parsley sprigs
1 orange

1. Brew the green tea and let cool.
2. Wash the dandelion greens, parsley, and orange.
3. Peel the orange and separate into sections.
4. Place a pitcher under the juicer's spout to collect the juice.
5. Feed the dandelion greens, parsley, and orange through the juicer's intake tube in the order listed.
6. When the juice stops flowing, remove the pitcher, add the green tea to the juice, and stir.
7. Serve immediately.

INGREDIENT TIP: Dandelion greens can be purchased at your local supermarket. But if you're using wild dandelions, make sure they are free of chemicals, such as pesticides, by washing them thoroughly.

PER SERVING: CALORIES: 61; TOTAL FAT: 1G; SUGAR: 9G; CARBOHYDRATES: 18G; FIBER: 1G; PROTEIN: 3G

MATCHA GREEN JUICE

Makes 1 (16-ounce) serving **Prep time:** 20 minutes

Matcha green tea has so many benefits. It boosts your metabolism and calms your mind. Matcha is full of antioxidants and detoxifies the body. You'll love how you feel after drinking this unique blend.

½ cup water
1 tsp matcha powder
4 green lettuce leaves
½ cucumber
½ lemon
½ green apple

1. Heat the water to 180°F. Whisk in the matcha powder and let cool.
2. Wash the lettuce, cucumber, lemon, and apple.
3. Trim the ends from the cucumber, then cut into 4-inch pieces.
4. Peel the lemon and cut into quarters.
5. Remove the apple core and discard. Cut the apple into quarters, leaving the peel intact.
6. Place a pitcher under the juicer's spout to collect the juice.
7. Feed the lettuce, cucumber, lemon, and apple through the juicer's intake tube in the order listed.
8. When the juice stops flowing, remove the pitcher, add the matcha mixture, and stir.
9. Serve immediately.

INGREDIENT TIP: Matcha powder should be very bright green in color. If it's not, the powder may have oxidized. To avoid this, buy matcha in small quantities and keep the container tightly sealed.

PER SERVING: CALORIES: 63; TOTAL FAT: 0G; SUGAR: 13G; CARBOHYDRATES: 20G; FIBER: 1G; PROTEIN: 1G

SPICED PEAR JUICE

Makes 1 (12-ounce) serving **Prep time:** 15 minutes

This juice reminds me of baked pears with cinnamon. Yum! The ingredients were chosen not only for their taste, but also for their ability to promote good health. Kale and turmeric help the body shed toxins and build the immune system. Pears aid healthy digestion. Lime improves the appearance of the skin, and cinnamon boosts energy and may accelerate weight loss.

6 kale leaves
2 pears
Fresh turmeric root
½ lime
½ teaspoon ground cinnamon

1. Wash the kale, pears, turmeric root, and lime.
2. Cut the pear into quarters, removing the core and seeds, but leaving the peel intact.
3. Slice off a 2-inch piece of the turmeric root.
4. Peel the lime and cut into quarters.
5. Place a pitcher under the juicer's spout to collect the juice.
6. Feed the first four ingredients through the juicer's intake tube in the order listed.
7. When the juice stops flowing, remove the pitcher, add the cinnamon, and stir the juice.
8. Serve immediately.

VARIATION TIP: Turn up the heat a notch by using just a pinch of cayenne pepper instead of cinnamon.

PER SERVING: CALORIES: 194; TOTAL FAT: 2G; SUGAR: 28G; CARBOHYDRATES: 58G; FIBER: 2G; PROTEIN: 8G

ASPARAGUS APPLE JUICE

Makes 1 (8-ounce) serving **Prep time:** 15 minutes

The taste of asparagus is earthy and bold, but also bright and clean when fresh. The soluble fiber in asparagus helps you feel full, making this vegetable beneficial for weight loss. Asparagus is a natural diuretic, too, which will help flush excess fluids from the body and may prevent urinary tract infections.

6 asparagus spears
1 green apple
2 celery ribs
¼ cup filtered water

1. Wash the asparagus, apple, and celery.
2. Trim ½ inch from the bottom of the asparagus, then cut stalks into 4-inch pieces.
3. Remove the apple core and discard. Cut the apple into quarters, leaving the peel intact.
4. Trim the ends from the celery, then cut into 4-inch pieces.
5. Place a pitcher under the juicer's spout to collect the juice.
6. Feed the asparagus, apple, and celery through the juicer's intake tube.
7. When the juice stops flowing, remove the pitcher, add the filtered water, and stir the juice.
8. Serve immediately.

PREPARATION TIP: To keep asparagus fresh before juicing, trim ½ inch from bottom of each stalk and place stalks, trimmed end down, in a widemouthed mason jar filled with an inch of water. Loosely cover the asparagus with a plastic bag and store in the refrigerator for up to 1 week.

PER SERVING: CALORIES: 61; TOTAL FAT: 0G; SUGAR: 13G; CARBOHYDRATES: 19G;

FIBER: 1G; PROTEIN: 2G

LOOKING GOOD, FEELING GOOD

Makes 1 (10-ounce) serving **Prep time:** 15 minutes

This juice is an all-around tonic that benefits your whole body and helps you shed weight more easily. Tomatoes, a good source of the antioxidant lycopene, help reduce the risk of heart disease and cancer. Carrots are beneficial for healthy, vibrant skin, and beets assist the liver in detoxifying the body.

---

1 bunch beet greens (5 to 6 stems)
1 green apple
1 cucumber
2 carrots
1 tomato
Fresh ginger root

1. Remove beet greens from beets.
2. Wash all the ingredients.
3. Remove the apple core and discard. Cut the apple into quarters, leaving the peel intact.
4. Trim the ends from the cucumber and carrots, then cut into 4-inch pieces.
5. Cut the tomato into quarters.
6. Slice off a 1-inch piece of the ginger root.
7. Place a pitcher under the juicer's spout to collect the juice.
8. Feed each ingredient through the juicer's intake tube in the order listed.
9. When the juice stops flowing, remove the pitcher and stir the juice.
10. Serve immediately.

INGREDIENT TIP: You can juice the green tops of beets and even put them in salads. The oxalic acid in these greens can be harmful when consumed in large amounts, but in small amounts, they are perfectly fine. Consult your doctor if you are concerned.

PER SERVING: CALORIES: 133; TOTAL FAT: 1G; SUGAR: 21G; CARBOHYDRATES: 42G; FIBER: 2G; PROTEIN: 6G

HEAVENLY DELIGHT

Makes 1 (10-ounce) serving **Prep time:** 15 minutes

Raspberries, coconut, and chocolate are a match made in heaven, and I was thrilled to find a way to use all three in a green juice recipe. Raw cacao, which is the purest form of chocolate, is a low-sugar and low-calorie ingredient that promotes weight loss and boosts immunity.

½ cup raspberries
4 kale leaves
½ red apple
1 cup coconut water
1 tablespoon raw cacao powder

1. Wash the raspberries, kale, and apple.
2. Remove the apple core and discard. Cut the apple into quarters, leaving the peel intact.
3. Place a pitcher under the juicer's spout to collect the juice.
4. Feed the raspberries, kale, and apple through the juicer's intake tube in the order listed.
5. When the juice stops flowing, remove the pitcher, add the coconut water and raw cacao powder, and stir the juice.
6. Serve immediately.

INGREDIENT TIP: Cacao and cocoa are both made from the same plant. Raw cacao, however, is made by cold-pressing unroasted cacao beans, and it contains living enzymes. Cocoa powder is raw cacao that's been roasted.

PER SERVING: CALORIES: 104; TOTAL FAT: 2G; SUGAR: 14G; CARBOHYDRATES: 27G; FIBER: 1G; PROTEIN: 6G

GREEN METAMORPHOSIS

Makes 1 (10-ounce) serving **Prep time:** 15 minutes

The best transformations occur simultaneously throughout the mind and body. The maca powder in this recipe benefits weight loss by helping control blood sugar levels, boost stamina, and regulate hormones. Maca also improves your mental ability to fight stress and anxiety.

---

2 cups mixed greens
1 orange
1 cucumber
½ lime
1 teaspoon maca powder

1. Wash the mixed greens, orange, cucumber, and lime.
2. Peel the orange and lime, then cut into quarters.
3. Trim the ends from the cucumber, then cut into 4-inch pieces.
4. Place a pitcher under the juicer's spout to collect the juice.
5. Feed the first four ingredients through the juicer's intake tube in the order listed.
6. When the juice stops flowing, remove the pitcher, add the maca powder, and stir the juice.
7. Serve immediately.

INGREDIENT TIP: Maca root is a powerful herb with a strong nutty flavor. Try beginning with ½ teaspoon until your body adjusts to this juice's flavor and benefits.

PER SERVING: CALORIES: 72; TOTAL FAT: 0G; SUGAR: 13G; CARBOHYDRATES: 22G; FIBER: 1G; PROTEIN: 3G

ENLIGHTEN ME JUICE

Makes 1 (10-ounce) serving **Prep time:** 15 minutes

Grapefruit is often included in weight loss diets because of its ability to help you feel full and burn fat. In a green juice, grapefruit becomes an essential part of a healthy morning routine. Some people find the taste bitter, but adding an apple will help offset the flavor.

2 cups spinach
½ grapefruit
4 celery ribs
½ apple
Fresh ginger root

1. Wash all the ingredients.
2. Peel the grapefruit and separate into sections.
3. Trim the ends from the celery, then cut into 4-inch pieces.
4. Remove the apple core and discard. Cut the apple into quarters, leaving the peel intact.
5. Slice off a 1-inch piece of the ginger root.
6. Place a pitcher under the juicer's spout to collect the juice.
7. Feed each ingredient through the juicer's intake tube in the order listed.
8. When the juice stops flowing, remove the pitcher and stir the juice.
9. Serve immediately.

INGREDIENT TIP: A ripe grapefruit should feel firm and look oval with a slightly flattened top and bottom. Avoid grapefruits that are lumpy or have an odd shape.

PER SERVING: CALORIES: 71; TOTAL FAT: 1G; SUGAR: 13G; CARBOHYDRATES: 22G; FIBER: 1G; PROTEIN: 3G

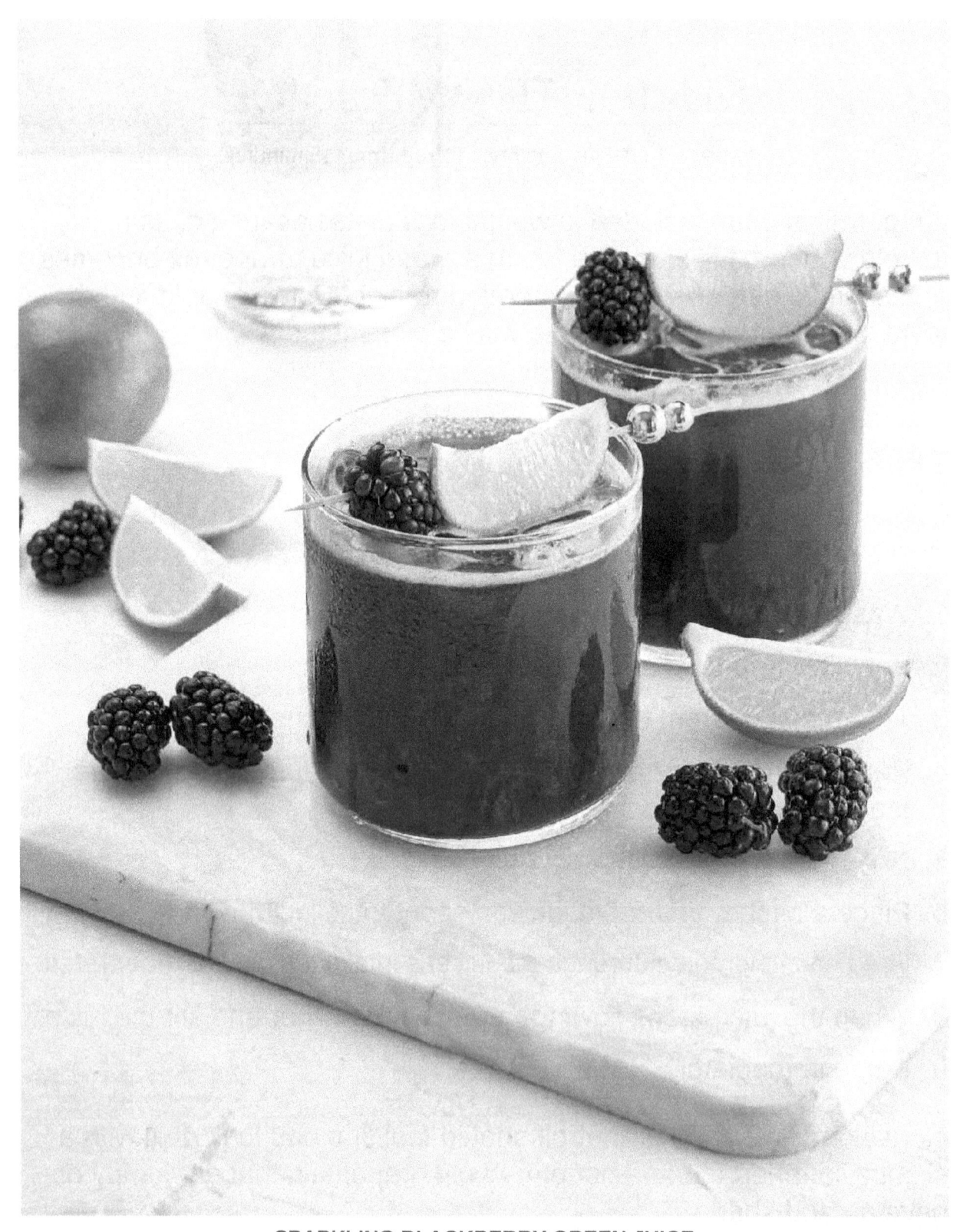

SPARKLING BLACKBERRY GREEN JUICE

5
Get Skin Glowing with Green

Royal Green

Green Healing Juice

Skin Detox Juice

Happy Face Green Juice

Angelica's Green Juice

Timeless Beauty Juice

Three Cheers for Kiwi

Clear Skin Juice

Sparkling Blackberry Green Juice

Antioxidant Supreme

Grapes and Greens

Tomatillo Green Mary

True beauty is a healthy glow that comes from the inside. Years ago, I made my own skin-care products with natural, pure ingredients. I used carrots, cucumbers, and various fruits to reduce inflammation, control sebum production, and brighten my skin tone. But when I began juicing, I realized that what you put into your body is what you get out of it. I knew I could achieve the same results by drinking the ingredients I had used in my skin-care treatments. I created the recipes in this chapter as tonics to promote great-looking skin, regardless of your skin type.

ROYAL GREEN

Makes 1 (12-ounce) serving **Prep time:** 10 minutes

With their high levels of antioxidants like copper and vitamins C and K, pears promote healthy complexions. Your skin loves antioxidants because they protect your body from potential free-radical damage. The simple ingredients in Royal Green juice are mild and palatable.

1 pear
3 cups baby spinach
1 cucumber ½
lemon Fresh
ginger root

1. Wash all the ingredients.
2. Cut the pear into quarters, removing the core and seeds, but leaving the peel intact.
3. Trim the ends from the cucumber, then cut into 4-inch pieces.
4. Peel the lemon and cut into quarters.
5. Slice off a ½-inch piece of the ginger root.
6. Place a pitcher under the juicer's spout to collect the juice.
7. Feed each ingredient through the juicer's intake tube in the order listed.
8. When the juice stops flowing, remove the pitcher and stir the juice.
9. Serve immediately.

VARIATION TIP: Cucumbers provide a wonderful way to cool and calm irritated skin. Pour some pure cucumber juice into a spray bottle and spritz on your face. Store in the refrigerator for up to 4 days.

PER SERVING: CALORIES: 135; TOTAL FAT: 1G; SUGAR: 21G; CARBOHYDRATES: 44G; FIBER: 1G; PROTEIN: 5G

GREEN HEALING JUICE

Makes 1 (12-ounce) serving **Prep time:** 15 minutes

The classic green juice is a blend of leafy greens that purify your cells. Cucumber hydrates, and herbs detoxify and brighten your appearance. My version contains half the fruit and twice the greens for a potent dose of healing energy.

---

2 cups spinach
3 kale leaves
½ cucumber
1 green apple
2 tablespoons cilantro sprigs
½ lime
Fresh ginger root

1. Wash all the ingredients.
2. Trim the ends from the cucumber, then cut into 4-inch pieces.
3. Remove the apple core and discard. Cut the apple into quarters, leaving the peel intact.
4. Peel the lime and cut into quarters.
5. Slice off a ½-inch piece of the ginger root.
6. Place a pitcher under the juicer's spout to collect the juice.
7. Feed each ingredient through the juicer's intake tube in the order listed.
8. When the juice stops flowing, remove the pitcher and stir the juice.
9. Serve immediately.

VARIATION TIP: Some people with a certain gene variation involved in sensing smells think that cilantro tastes like soap. If this is you, feel free to substitute curly parsley for cilantro in recipes.

PER SERVING: CALORIES: 103; TOTAL FAT: 1G; SUGAR: 16G; CARBOHYDRATES: 31G; FIBER: 1G; PROTEIN: 4G

SKIN DETOX JUICE

Makes 1 (12-ounce) serving **Prep time:** 15 minutes

Orange foods, like sweet potatoes, are high in beta-carotene and help combat rough and dry skin. The greens in this juice help your body detox. Antioxidants in zucchini protect skin cells from premature aging, lighten the skin, and improve the overall health of skin, hair, and nails. You can drink this rich, sweet juice as a part of your regular beauty routine.

---

1 cup spinach
1 cup cubed sweet potato
3 celery ribs
1 zucchini
1 cucumber
½ lemon

1. Wash all the ingredients.
2. Peel the sweet potato and cut into small cubes.
3. Trim the ends from the celery, zucchini, and cucumber, then cut into 4-inch pieces.
4. Peel the lemon half and cut into quarters.
5. Place a pitcher under the juicer's spout to collect the juice.
6. Feed each ingredient through the juicer's intake tube in the order listed.
7. When the juice stops flowing, remove the pitcher and stir the juice.
8. Serve immediately.

BEAUTY TIP: Buy an extra sweet potato to make a conditioner for dry hair. Peel and boil the potato, then mash it up with 1 cup yogurt and 1 tablespoon honey. Apply to hair for 15 minutes, then rinse.

PER SERVING: CALORIES: 123; TOTAL FAT: 1G; SUGAR: 11G; CARBOHYDRATES: 34G; FIBER: 1G; PROTEIN: 5G

HAPPY FACE GREEN JUICE

Makes 1 (12-ounce) serving **Prep time:** 15 minutes

I've had issues with acne off and on since my teenage years. These days, I know I can use food to support my skin and clear up my face. I turn to carrots to promote an even skin tone and turmeric root for its anti-inflammatory and antibacterial benefits.

6 carrots
1 romaine heart
2 celery ribs
1 orange
Fresh ginger root
Fresh turmeric root

1. Wash all the ingredients.
2. Trim the ends from the carrots and celery, then cut into 4-inch pieces.
3. Peel the orange and cut into quarters.
4. Slice off ½-inch pieces of the ginger root and the turmeric root.
5. Place a pitcher under the juicer's spout to collect the juice.
6. Feed each ingredient through the juicer's intake tube in the order listed.
7. When the juice stops flowing, remove the pitcher and stir the juice.
8. Serve immediately.

BEAUTY TIP: Carrot pulp makes a great facial mask for any skin type. Add 3 to 4 tablespoons of honey to ¼ cup carrot pulp and apply to your face. Leave on for 10 minutes, then rinse. If the paste is too thick, add 1 to 2 teaspoons of carrot juice.

PER SERVING: CALORIES: 151; TOTAL FAT: 2G; SUGAR: 24G; CARBOHYDRATES: 46G; FIBER: 2G; PROTEIN: 7G

ANGELICA'S GREEN JUICE

Makes 1 (8-ounce) serving **Prep time:** 15 minutes

This juice is named after a friend who has the most gorgeous hair and glowing skin. For this recipe, I've combined strawberries and kale, two antioxidant-rich foods that promote cellular regeneration and detoxification.

---

6 strawberries
6 kale leaves
2 celery ribs
½ cucumber

1. Wash all the ingredients.
2. Trim the ends from the celery and cucumber, then cut into 4-inch pieces.
3. Place a pitcher under the juicer's spout to collect the juice.
4. Feed each ingredient through the juicer's intake tube in the order listed.
5. When the juice stops flowing, remove the pitcher and stir the juice.
6. Serve immediately.

PREPARATION TIP: You don't have to remove the greens from your strawberries. Just be sure to clean off any dirt completely.

PER SERVING: CALORIES: 84; TOTAL FAT: 2G; SUGAR: 8G; CARBOHYDRATES: 22G; FIBER: 1G; PROTEIN: 8G

TIMELESS BEAUTY JUICE

Makes 1 (8-ounce) serving **Prep time:** 20 minutes

The small amount of extra time it takes to make this juice is worth the effort. Artichokes contribute to healthy collagen development and the appearance of younger-looking skin. For that reason, you'll often find artichoke extract in luxury skin-care products.

1 artichoke
1 green apple
1 cup spinach
1 celery rib

1. Wash all the ingredients.
2. Prepare the artichoke per the instructions in the Preparation Tip.
3. Remove the apple core and discard. Cut the apple into quarters, leaving the peel intact.
4. Trim the ends from the celery, then cut into 4-inch pieces.
5. Place a pitcher under the juicer's spout to collect the juice. Then, feed each ingredient through the juicer's intake tube in the order listed.
6. When the juice stops flowing, remove the pitcher and stir the juice.
7. Serve immediately.

PREPARATION TIP: It's easy to prepare an artichoke for this recipe.

1. Slice the stem from the artichoke and cut it into small pieces.
2. Trim 1 to 2 inches off the top.
3. Press down on the center to open the leaves.
4. Rinse well under running water.
5. Scoop out the hairy center with a grapefruit spoon.

6. Tear or cut away the leaves.

7. Place into a food processor or blender and process until the consistency is even.

PER SERVING: CALORIES: 75; TOTAL FAT: 0G; SUGAR: 12G; CARBOHYDRATES: 25G; FIBER: 1G; PROTEIN: 4G

THREE CHEERS FOR KIWI

Makes 1 (16-ounce) serving **Prep time:** 15 minutes

The bright green color of this juice will delight your eyes as much as its sweet yet slightly tart flavor appeals to your taste buds. Kiwis are popular fruit, known for their ability to firm skin, control excess sebum production, lighten dark circles, and prevent premature gray hair.

4 kiwis
4 cups spinach
1 cucumber
1 lime
Pinch sea salt

1. Wash the kiwis, spinach, cucumber, and lime.
2. Trim the ends from the cucumber, then cut into 4-inch pieces.
3. Peel the kiwis and lime and cut them into quarters.
4. Place a pitcher under the juicer's spout to collect the juice.
5. Feed the first four ingredients through the juicer's intake tube in the order listed.
6. When the juice stops flowing, remove the pitcher, add the sea salt, and stir the juice.
7. Serve immediately.

INGREDIENT TIP: Sea salt contains trace elements of vital minerals such as potassium, magnesium, and calcium. In green juice, sea salt serves to balance out tart flavors.

PER SERVING: CALORIES: 145; TOTAL FAT: 2G; SUGAR: 22G; CARBOHYDRATES: 43G; FIBER: 1G; PROTEIN: 6G

CLEAR SKIN JUICE

Makes 1 (12-ounce) serving **Prep time:** 15 minutes

Each ingredient in this recipe promotes healthy skin. Carrots boost collagen production. Lemons brighten skin, while broccoli provides a healthy glow. Turmeric root reduces redness and inflammation, and the detoxifying mustard greens add a spicy kick.

---

8 carrots
4 mustard green leaves
3 lemons
2 cups broccoli
Fresh turmeric root

1. Wash all the ingredients.
2. Trim the ends from the carrots, then cut into 4-inch pieces.
3. Peel the lemons and cut into quarters.
4. Remove the stalk from the broccoli crown with a knife and discard or save to juice later. Cut the crown into small florets.
5. Slice off a 2-inch piece of the turmeric root.
6. Place a pitcher under the juicer's spout to collect the juice.
7. Feed each ingredient through the juicer's intake tube in the order listed.
8. When the juice stops flowing, remove the pitcher and stir the juice.
9. Serve immediately.

INGREDIENT TIP: You can choose from many varieties of mustard greens, from curly to flat in shape and green to purple in color. In the spring, you also may notice that the leaves of mustard greens are smaller and more tender.

PER SERVING: CALORIES: 171; TOTAL FAT: 2G; SUGAR: 22G; CARBOHYDRATES: 55G;

FIBER: 3G; PROTEIN: 9G

SPARKLING BLACKBERRY GREEN JUICE

Makes 1 (12-ounce) serving **Prep time:** 10 minutes

As you drink this juice, close your eyes and imagine yourself at a spa, sipping on a healing elixir. The blackberries help your body reduce inflammation and fight infections, while the collard greens encourage a youthful glow.

½ cup blackberries
4 large collard green leaves
½ lime
8 ounces sparkling mineral water

1. Wash the blackberries, collard greens, and lime.
2. Peel the lime and cut into quarters.
3. Feed the first three ingredients through the juicer's intake tube in the order listed.
4. When the juice stops flowing, remove the pitcher, add the mineral water, and stir the juice.
5. Serve immediately.

INGREDIENT TIP: The peak season for blackberries is late summer. You can stock up on these beauties when they are on sale, put them in the freezer, and then thaw them before use.

PER SERVING: CALORIES: 30; TOTAL FAT: 1G; SUGAR: 3G; CARBOHYDRATES: 12G; FIBER: 1G; PROTEIN: 3G

ANTIOXIDANT SUPREME

Makes 1 (12-ounce) serving **Prep time:** 15 minutes

If you think all green juices taste the same, think again. This juice has an exotic yet mellow flavor. Blackberries give this recipe an incredible dark green color, while the fennel adds a flavorful twist.

4 kale leaves
½ cup blackberries
½ green apple
1 cup broccoli
1 cucumber ½

fennel bulb

1. Wash all the ingredients.
2. Remove the apple core and discard. Cut the apple into quarters, leaving the peel intact.
3. Remove the stalk from the broccoli crown with a knife and discard or save to juice later. Cut the crown into small florets.
4. Trim the ends from the cucumber, then cut into 4-inch pieces.
5. Remove the stalks and fronds from the fennel and save for later. Cut the bulb into quarters.
6. Place a pitcher under the juicer's spout to collect the juice.
7. Feed each ingredient through the juicer's intake tube in the order listed.
8. When the juice stops flowing, remove the pitcher and stir the juice.
9. Serve immediately.

INGREDIENT TIP: Save your fennel stalks and fronds. Think of fennel fronds (the leafy parts) as herbs and use them in salads, in marinades, in soups, or with meats. You can substitute the stalks for celery in most recipes.

PER SERVING: CALORIES: 138; TOTAL FAT: 2G; SUGAR: 18G; CARBOHYDRATES: 41G; FIBER: 2G; PROTEIN: 10G

GRAPES AND GREENS

Makes 1 (12-ounce) serving **Prep time:** 15 minutes

Grapes are fun to use in juicing because they don't need to be peeled or cut, and they produce a large quantity of juice. This straightforward recipe brims with good ingredients that will make your skin feel hydrated and supple.

---

3 Swiss chard leaves
3 romaine lettuce leaves
1 cup green grapes
1½ cucumbers

1. Wash all the ingredients.
2. Trim the ends from the cucumbers, then cut into 4-inch pieces.
3. Place a pitcher under the juicer's spout to collect the juice.
4. Feed each ingredient through the juicer's intake tube in the order listed.
5. When the juice stops flowing, remove the pitcher and stir the juice.
6. Serve immediately.

BEAUTY TIP: Have extra grapes from juicing? Use them to nourish your fingernails. Cut 5 grapes in half and dip the fleshy side in granulated sugar. Rub a grape half over each nail, including the cuticle. Wipe away sugar and massage each nail with a drop of grapeseed oil.

PER SERVING: CALORIES: 128; TOTAL FAT: 1G; SUGAR: 23G; CARBOHYDRATES: 36G; FIBER: 1G; PROTEIN: 5G

TOMATILLO GREEN MARY

Makes 1 (16-ounce) serving **Prep time:** 20 minutes

This is a healthy and nonalcoholic green version of the Bloody Mary drink. This drink is a little spicy, but the pineapple juice cools it down and helps your body fight skin damage caused by the sun and pollution. Your skin also will love how the vitamin C content from the pineapple and jalapeño helps heal tissues and wounds.

2 tomatillos
1 cucumber
¼ cup cilantro sprigs
2 celery ribs
½ jalapeño pepper
½ lime
½ cup pineapple juice

1. Wash all the produce.
2. Peel the outer leaf away from the tomatillos, then cut into quarters.
3. Trim the ends from the cucumber and celery, then cut into 4-inch pieces.
4. Remove the stem and seeds from the jalapeño.
5. Peel the lime and cut into quarters.
6. Place a pitcher under the juicer's spout to collect the juice.
7. Feed the first six ingredients through the juicer's intake tube in the order listed.
8. When the juice stops flowing, remove the pitcher, add the pineapple juice, and stir.
9. Serve immediately.

DID YOU KNOW? The enzyme bromelain, which is found in pineapples, does more than break down foods in your digestive tract. When used externally on the skin, the enzyme is a gentle exfoliant that cleanses and removes dead skin cells.

PER SERVING: CALORIES: 119; TOTAL FAT: 1G; SUGAR: 13G; CARBOHYDRATES: 16G; FIBER: 7G; PROTEIN: 4G

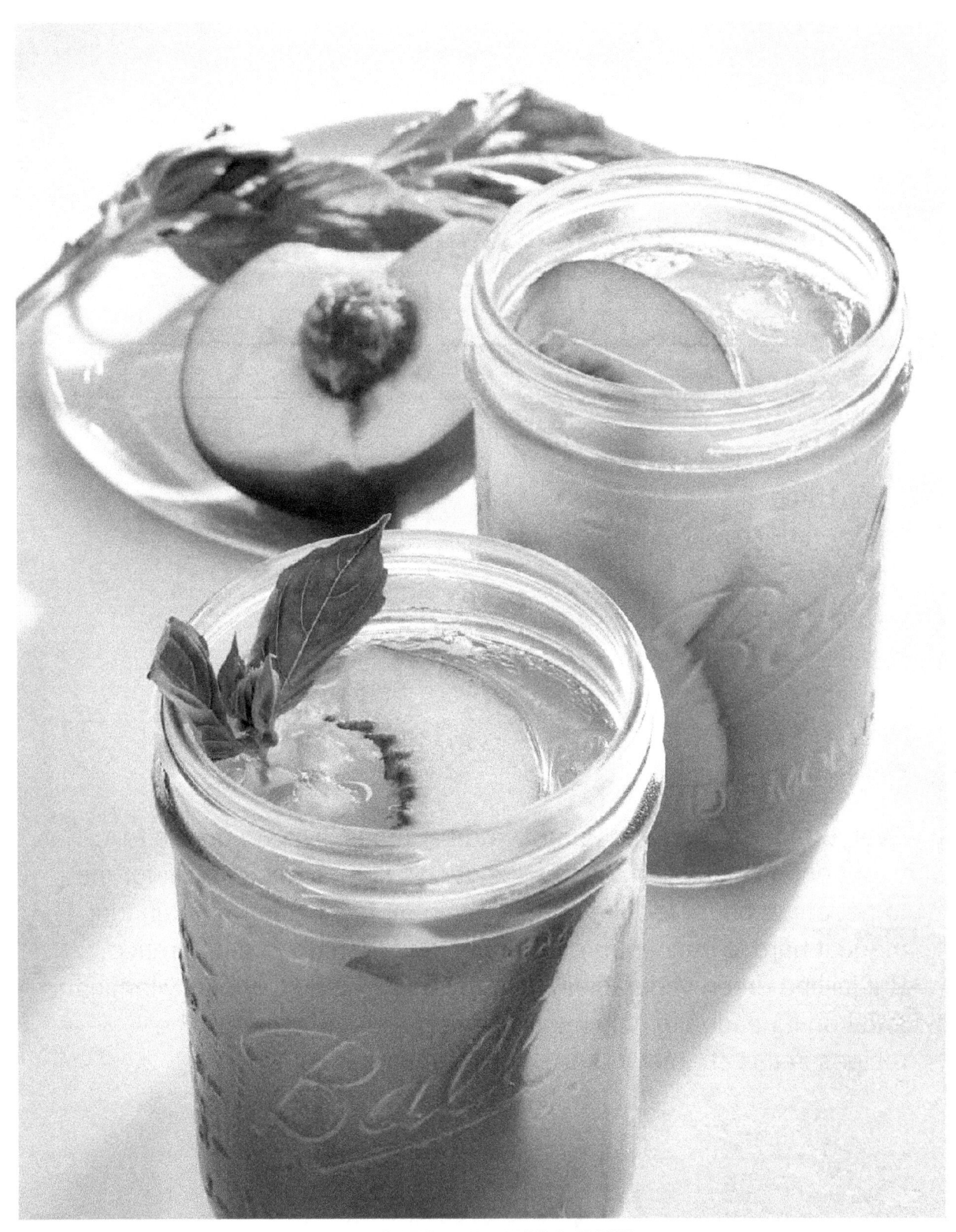

PEACHES AND HERBS JUICE

6
Energize with Green

Electrolyte Power Juice

Wheatgrass Supreme

Seize the Day

Get Your Juice On

Green Extreme

Green Protein Power

Juice of Champions

Daily Endurance Juice

Peaches and Herbs Juice

Motivate Me

Make My Day Juice

Stay Rad Green Juice

Everyone feels tired and unmotivated at times. When I began to experience fatigue in my early 30s, it was sometimes difficult for me to get out of bed. I felt like I had a constant fog inside my brain that made it hard to concentrate. Exercise and rest made a difference. But juicing green vegetables gave my body the supply of B vitamins and iron it needed to help me feel energized and upbeat. The recipes in this chapter will get you up and running, too.

ELECTROLYTE POWER JUICE

Makes 1 (16-ounce) serving **Prep time:** 10 minutes

Electrolytes are necessary for the proper functioning of the digestive, cardiac, nervous, and muscular systems. Electrolytes contain calcium, potassium, sodium, and magnesium to hydrate your cells so that everything runs smoothly. Skip the premade electrolyte drinks that contain added sugar and go with this fresh green juice instead.

2 cups spinach
6 celery ribs
1 cup blueberries
8 ounces coconut water

1. Wash the spinach, celery, and blueberries.
2. Trim the ends from the celery, then cut into 4-inch pieces.
3. Place a pitcher under the juicer's spout to collect the juice.
4. Feed the first three ingredients through the juicer's intake tube in the order listed.
5. When the juice stops flowing, remove the pitcher, add the coconut water, and stir.
6. Serve immediately.

VARIATION TIP: To try a variety of flavors, swap out the blueberries for strawberries, cherries, or watermelon. Berries are high in vitamins A and C, making them great for heart health. Watermelon contains thiamine, vitamin B6, and folate, all of which help boost your energy.

PER SERVING: CALORIES: 73; TOTAL FAT: 1G; SUGAR: 13G; CARBOHYDRATES: 21G; FIBER: 1G; PROTEIN: 3G

WHEATGRASS SUPREME

Makes 1 (12-ounce) serving **Prep time:** 15 minutes

Wheatgrass has a powerful, earthy flavor that does, in fact, taste like grass. That might not sound appealing, but the orange in this recipe makes the juice sweeter. Adding wheatgrass to your diet is a great idea because it is one of the best sources of chlorophyll, which supports the purification of your blood.

1 cucumber
2 cups spinach
1 handful wheatgrass
1 orange
1 green apple

1. Wash all the ingredients.
2. Trim the ends from the cucumber, then cut into 4-inch pieces.
3. Peel the orange and cut into quarters.
4. Remove the apple core and discard. Cut the apple into quarters, leaving the peel intact.
5. Place a pitcher under the juicer's spout to collect the juice.
6. Feed each ingredient through the juicer's intake tube in the order listed.
7. When the juice stops flowing, remove the pitcher and stir the juice.
8. Serve immediately.

INGREDIENT TIP: Wheatgrass, a young sprouted grass, does not contain gluten, though it is a type of wheat plant. Gluten is found only in the seed kernels of the wheat plant.

PER SERVING: CALORIES: 133; TOTAL FAT: 1G; SUGAR: 23G; CARBOHYDRATES: 34G; FIBER: 1G; PROTEIN: 6G

SEIZE THE DAY

Makes 1 (12-ounce) serving **Prep time:** 20 minutes

Can't decide between green juice, green tea, or a morning fiber drink? Why not choose them all? Spinach in this 3-for-1 juice provides antioxidants, green tea gives you energy, and flax seed supports a healthy digestive tract. The texture is a bit thick due to the ground flax seeds, but the seeds won't affect the taste.

¾ cup green tea
2 cups spinach 1
red apple
2 teaspoons ground flax seed

1. Brew the green tea and let it cool.
2. Wash the spinach and apple.
3. Remove the apple core and discard. Cut the apple into quarters, leaving the peel intact.
4. Place a pitcher under the juicer's spout to collect the juice.
5. Feed the spinach, then the apple through the juicer's intake tube.
6. When the juice stops flowing, remove the pitcher, add the green tea and flax seed, then stir.
7. Serve immediately.

INGREDIENT TIP: Because flax seed contains a high amount of oil, ground flax seed can spoil quickly—in as little as a week. It's best to buy whole seeds and use a spice or coffee grinder to grind only what you need.

PER SERVING: CALORIES: 66; TOTAL FAT: 2G; SUGAR: 11G; CARBOHYDRATES: 17G; FIBER: 1G; PROTEIN: 2G

GET YOUR JUICE ON

Makes 1 (12-ounce) serving **Prep time:** 15 minutes

This juice is perfect if you're a little reluctant to take the leap into green juicing. This drink has a subtle green appearance with flavors so well balanced that you won't realize you're drinking parsley, an herb with a strong flavor that detoxifies the blood, liver, and kidneys.

2 cucumbers
3 carrots
2 tablespoons parsley
1 sprig mint leaves
Fresh ginger root

1. Wash all the ingredients.
2. Trim the ends from the cucumbers and carrots, then cut into 4-inch pieces.
3. Slice off a ½-inch piece of the ginger root.
4. Place a pitcher under the juicer's spout to collect the juice.
5. Feed each ingredient through the juicer's intake tube in the order listed.
6. When the juice stops flowing, remove the pitcher and stir the juice.
7. Serve immediately.

INGREDIENT TIP: There are two kinds of parsley: curly, flat, and Italian. Try the curly variety first if you are new to eating greens. The curly variety has a milder flavor than Italian parsley.

PER SERVING: CALORIES: 94; TOTAL FAT: 1G; SUGAR: 11G; CARBOHYDRATES: 26G; FIBER: 1G; PROTEIN: 4G

GREEN EXTREME

Makes 1 (16-ounce) serving **Prep time:** 15 minutes

This green juice uses very little fruit, and it's extreme because every ingredient is green. Chances are, it'll make you feel like you can take on the world.

---

1 cucumber
1 romaine heart
4 celery ribs
1 lime
½ tablespoon wheatgrass powder

1. Wash the cucumber, romaine, celery, and lime.
2. Trim the ends from the cucumber and celery, then cut into 4-inch pieces.
3. Peel the lime and cut into quarters.
4. Place a pitcher under the juicer's spout to collect the juice.
5. Feed the first four ingredients through the juicer's intake tube in the order listed.
6. When the juice stops flowing, remove the pitcher, add the wheatgrass powder, and stir the juice.
7. Serve immediately.

DID YOU KNOW? Wheatgrass has been known to soothe menstrual pain, which can be worsened by vitamin and mineral deficiencies. A daily shot of fresh wheatgrass juice (alone or in combination with other greens) is highly nourishing and supports your body's natural detoxification process.

PER SERVING: CALORIES: 98; TOTAL FAT: 1G; SUGAR: 8G; CARBOHYDRATES: 26G; FIBER: 2G; PROTEIN: 7G

GREEN PROTEIN POWER

Makes 1 (14-ounce) serving **Prep time:** 15 minutes

After a workout, you need a healthy treat that will provide hydration, improve your recovery, and enhance your performance. Kale and chard leaves contain protein, and you can add your own protein powder to this juice for an extra boost.

---

1 cup pineapple
5 kale leaves
3 chard leaves
1 cucumber
2 scoops plant-based protein powder

1. Wash the kale, chard, and cucumber.
2. Trim the ends and skin from the pineapple, then remove the core and discard. Cut pineapple into 1-inch chunks.
3. Trim the ends from the cucumber, then cut into 4-inch pieces.
4. Place a pitcher under the juicer's spout to collect the juice.
5. Feed the first four ingredients through the juicer's intake tube in the order listed.
6. When the juice stops flowing, remove the pitcher, add the protein powder, and stir.
7. Serve immediately.

INGREDIENT TIP: When choosing a protein powder, make sure protein is the first ingredient listed on the label. It's also a good idea to select a brand with the lowest amount of added sugar.

PER SERVING: CALORIES: 335; TOTAL FAT: 6G; SUGAR: 19G; CARBOHYDRATES: 37G; FIBER: 1G; PROTEIN: 49G

JUICE OF CHAMPIONS

Makes 1 (12-ounce) serving **Prep time:** 15 minutes

This hearty juice is both flavorful and good for your heart. Beets contain high levels of antioxidants and other vitamins that help lower blood pressure, boost endurance, and fight cancer. Beets also help boost immunity.

1 cucumber
1 Swiss chard leaf
2 sprigs cilantro
½ small to medium size beet
3 celery ribs
½ lemon
Fresh ginger root

1. Wash all the ingredients.
2. Trim the ends from the cucumber and celery, then cut into 4-inch pieces.
3. Remove any greens from the beet and save for juicing later. Cut the beet into quarters.
4. Peel the lemon and cut into quarters.
5. Slice off a 1-inch piece of the ginger root.
6. Place a pitcher under the juicer's spout to collect the juice.
7. Feed each ingredient through the juicer's intake tube in the order listed.
8. When the juice stops flowing, remove the pitcher and stir the juice.
9. Serve immediately.

HEALTH TIP: Many heart-shaped fruits and vegetables are truly good for your heart. That's another good reason to consider choosing beets, tomatoes, apples, and strawberries the next time you buy fruits and vegetables.

PER SERVING: CALORIES: 76; TOTAL FAT: 1G; SUGAR: 10G; CARBOHYDRATES: 22G; FIBER: 1G; PROTEIN: 4G

DAILY ENDURANCE JUICE

Makes 1 (16-ounce) serving **Prep time:** 15 minutes

Broccoli packs a punch in this juice that has nearly 270 percent of your daily vitamin C requirements. Broccoli also contains about 3 grams of protein per cup. Many athletes choose this vegetable because it contains the nutrients needed to enhance tissue growth and heal the body.

2 cups broccoli
2 cucumbers
1 green apple
2 mint sprigs

1. Wash all the ingredients.
2. Remove the stalk from the broccoli crown with a knife and discard or save to juice later. Cut the crown into small florets.
3. Trim the ends from the cucumber, then cut into 4-inch pieces.
4. Remove the apple core and discard. Cut the apple into quarters, leaving the peel intact.
5. Place a pitcher under the juicer's spout to collect the juice.
6. Feed each ingredient through the juicer's intake tube in the order listed.
7. When the juice stops flowing, remove the pitcher and stir the juice.
8. Serve immediately.

INGREDIENT TIP: Don't throw out those broccoli stems. Their nutritional value is nearly identical to that of the crown, and they taste even sweeter. The stems can be juiced or used in other recipes like broccoli-stem pesto.

PER SERVING: CALORIES: 152; TOTAL FAT: 1G; SUGAR: 21G; CARBOHYDRATES: 43G; FIBER: 2G; PROTEIN: 9G

PEACHES AND HERBS JUICE

Makes 1 (8-ounce) serving **Prep time:** 15 minutes

Calling all adventurous souls! The delightful, herbaceous flavors of peach and basil in this green juice are sure to fulfill your desire for something different. The featured nutrient is iron, which boosts energy and improves brain and muscle health.

2 celery ribs
1 peach
5 basil leaves
2 chard leaves
½ lemon
¼ cup aloe vera juice

1. Wash all the produce.
2. Remove the peach pit and discard. Cut the peach into quarters, leaving the peel intact.
3. Peel the lemon half and cut into quarters.
4. Place a pitcher under the juicer's spout to collect the juice.
5. Feed the first five ingredients through the juicer's intake tube in the order listed.
6. When the juice stops flowing, remove the pitcher, add the aloe vera juice, and stir.
7. Serve immediately.

DID YOU KNOW? You can grow your own basil without dirt. All you need is a healthy basil stem and a glass of clean water. Remove the lower leaves and place the stem in the water glass in a location where it will receive sunlight.

PER SERVING: CALORIES: 101; TOTAL FAT: 1G; SUGAR: 18G; CARBOHYDRATES: 26G; FIBER: 1G; PROTEIN: 3G

MOTIVATE ME

Makes 1 (10-ounce) serving **Prep time:** 15 minutes

Thick and dark green, this unusual-looking juice tastes like a blueberry dessert, only it's much healthier. Maca reportedly helps you gain muscle, increases strength, boosts energy, and improves physical performance. Motivation? Check!

1 cup blueberries
2 cups spinach
1 cucumber Fresh
ginger root
½ teaspoon maca powder
¼ teaspoon cinnamon

1. Wash the blueberries, spinach, cucumber, and ginger root.
2. Trim the ends from the cucumber, then cut into 4-inch pieces.
3. Slice off a ½-inch piece of the ginger root.
4. Place a pitcher under the juicer's spout to collect the juice.
5. Feed the first four ingredients through the juicer's intake tube in the order listed.
6. When the juice stops flowing, remove the pitcher, add the maca powder and cinnamon, then stir.
7. Serve immediately.

DID YOU KNOW? A cinnamon tree can grow up to 60 feet tall. The spice you eat comes from the bark.

PER SERVING: CALORIES: 95; TOTAL FAT: 1G; SUGAR: 14G; CARBOHYDRATES: 27G; FIBER: 1G; PROTEIN: 4G

MAKE MY DAY JUICE

Makes 1 (12-ounce) serving **Prep time:** 15 minutes

This sweet and refreshing juice will make your day. The mint stimulates your mind, the kale detoxifies your body, and the oranges and carrots keep you looking and feeling vibrant.

2 oranges
5 carrots
½ lemon
8 kale leaves
15 mint leaves

1. Wash all the ingredients.
2. Peel the oranges and lemon, then cut into quarters.
3. Trim the ends from the carrots, then cut into 4-inch pieces.
4. Place a pitcher under the juicer's spout to collect the juice.
5. Feed each ingredient through the juicer's intake tube in the order listed.
6. When the juice stops flowing, remove the pitcher and stir the juice.
7. Serve immediately.

VARIATION TIP: Want to perk up the flavor with a different herb? Try fresh rosemary instead of mint.

PER SERVING: CALORIES: 210; TOTAL FAT: 3G; SUGAR: 32G; CARBOHYDRATES: 61G; FIBER: 3G; PROTEIN: 12G

STAY RAD GREEN JUICE

Makes 1 (12-ounce) serving **Prep time:** 15 minutes

Radishes are known to promote weight loss, lower blood pressure, and protect the immune system. They also add a little tang to a green juice. Drink this to put a kick in your step for the day.

2 cups spinach
1 head leaf lettuce (about 12 leaves)
10 sprigs cilantro
12 carrots
2 radishes
½ lemon

1. Wash all the ingredients.
2. Trim the ends from the carrots, then cut into 4-inch pieces.
3. Remove the tops from radishes.
4. Peel the lemon and cut into quarters.
5. Place a pitcher under the juicer's spout to collect the juice.
6. Feed each ingredient through the juicer's intake tube in the order listed.
7. When the juice stops flowing, remove the pitcher and stir the juice.
8. Serve immediately.

INGREDIENT TIP: Radishes have distinct tastes depending on their variety and where they were grown. If you previously passed on radishes because they were too spicy, try a different kind. You might find one or more you like.

PER SERVING: CALORIES: 186; TOTAL FAT: 2G; SUGAR: 26G; CARBOHYDRATES: 56G; FIBER: 3G; PROTEIN: 9G

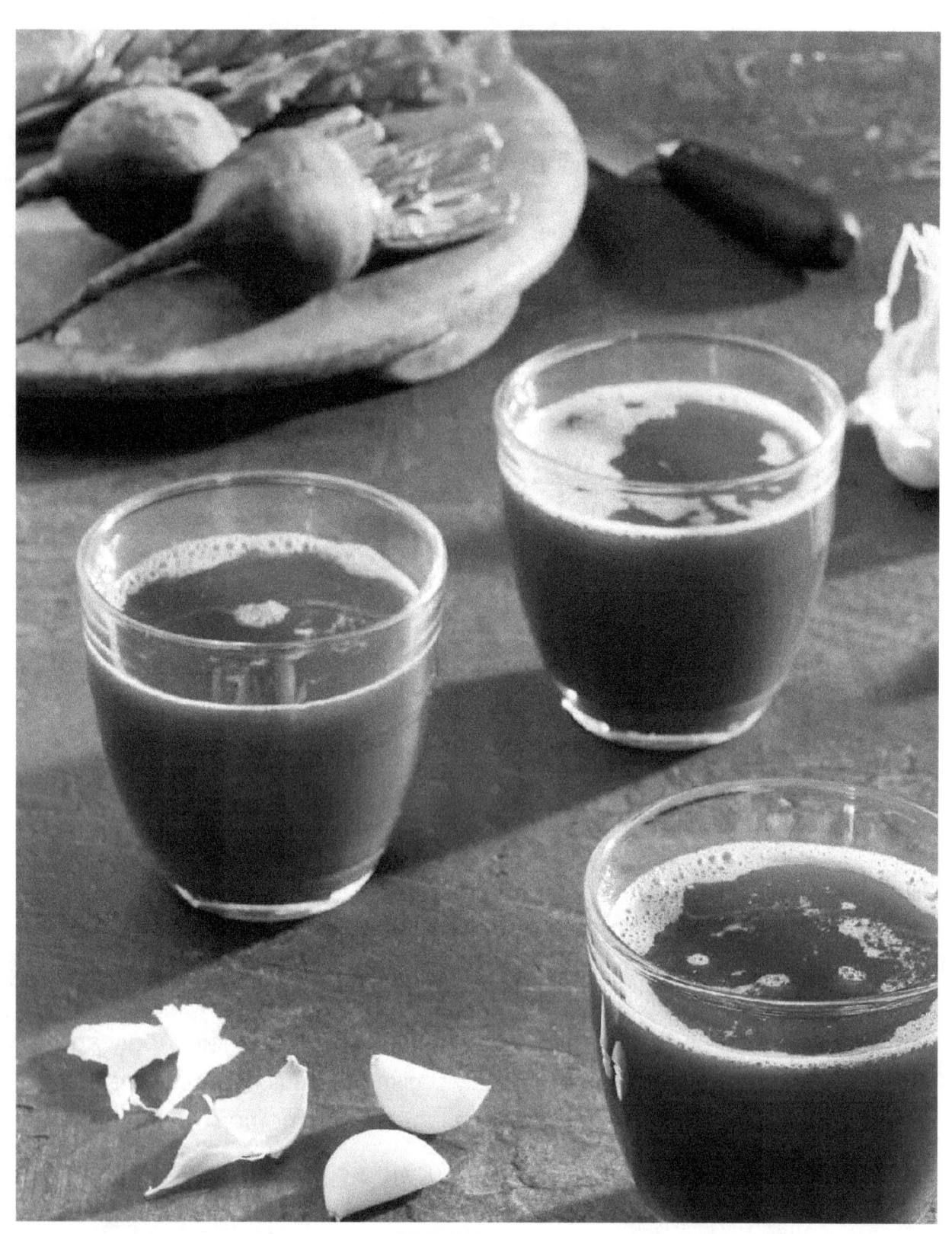

IMMUNITY PLUS

7
Green Immunity

Down to Earth Juice

Ulcer Care

Anti-Inflammatory Juice

Simple Detox Juice

Greens 'n' Garlic

Cleanse Assist

Ginger Blast

Immunity Plus

Aloe Cleanser

Good, Good, Good Digestion

Vitamin C Celebration

Healthy Healing Greens

"Treat your body well because without your body, where are you going to live?" That wisdom comes from a health-coach friend, and I think of it often because it's so true. We live in a world that frequently exposes us to chemicals and synthetic foods. We're stressed out by daily demands and the pressure to be productive. No wonder so many people experience chronic pain, poor digestion, and heart disease, not to mention colds, flus, and headaches. The recipes in this chapter target specific ailments and provide general healing for your mind and body.

DOWN TO EARTH JUICE

Makes 1 (12-ounce) serving **Prep time:** 15 minutes

The best word to describe cabbage juice is "earthy." Cabbage is rich in soluble fiber, which increases the beneficial bacteria in the gut. The apples in this recipe add a sweetness you'll appreciate.

½ cup cabbage
3 celery ribs
1 cucumber
1 cup spinach
2 apples

1. Wash all the ingredients.
2. Cut the cabbage in half, then slice or chop one half into smaller pieces.
3. Trim the ends from the celery and cucumber, then cut into 4-inch pieces.
4. Remove the apple cores and discard. Cut the apples into quarters, leaving the peel intact.
5. Place a pitcher under the juicer's spout to collect the juice.
6. Feed each ingredient through the juicer's intake tube in the order listed.
7. When the juice stops flowing, remove the pitcher and stir the juice.
8. Serve immediately.

DID YOU KNOW? Cabbage is a great source of vitamin K1, providing 85 percent of your daily recommendation in 1 cup.

PER SERVING: CALORIES: 132; TOTAL FAT: 1G; SUGAR: 27G; CARBOHYDRATES: 41G; FIBER: 1G; PROTEIN: 3G

ULCER CARE

Makes 1 (12-ounce) serving **Prep time:** 15 minutes

Greens are beneficial for your digestion and gut health. Cabbage juice in particular has long been used as a home remedy for ulcers. Its natural glutamine is believed to nourish and repair the gut lining, but if you have a medical condition, be sure to check with your doctor first.

---

2 cups green cabbage
2 cups spinach
3 green chard leaves
3 celery ribs
1 green apple

1. Wash all the ingredients.
2. Cut the cabbage in half, then slice or chop into smaller pieces.
3. Trim the ends from the celery, then cut into 4-inch pieces.
4. Remove the apple core and discard. Cut the apple into quarters, leaving the peel intact.
5. Place a pitcher under the juicer's spout to collect the juice.
6. Feed each ingredient through the juicer's intake tube in the order listed.
7. When the juice stops flowing, remove the pitcher and stir the juice.
8. Serve immediately.

VARIATION TIP: There are many varieties of cabbage, each with a slightly different flavor. Red or purple cabbage has a deeper flavor. Napa cabbage, an oblong-shaped cabbage, tastes crisper and sweeter than green cabbage. Savoy cabbage is dark green and has a mild flavor.

PER SERVING: CALORIES: 88; TOTAL FAT: 1G; SUGAR: 16G; CARBOHYDRATES: 28G; FIBER: 1G; PROTEIN: 5G

ANTI-INFLAMMATORY JUICE

Makes 1 (12-ounce) serving **Prep time:** 15 minutes

Research shows that chronic inflammation is likely a common factor in heart disease and autoimmune disorders. The ingredients in this juice, which contains vitamin K and antioxidants, protect against oxidative stress and help reduce inflammation.

1 cup spinach
4 carrots
2 celery ribs
1 green apple
½ teaspoon ground cinnamon

1. Wash the spinach, carrots, celery, and apple.
2. Trim the ends from the carrots and celery, then cut into 4-inch pieces.
3. Remove the apple core and discard. Cut the apple into quarters, leaving the peel intact.
4. Place a pitcher under the juicer's spout to collect the juice.
5. Feed the first four ingredients through the juicer's intake tube in the order listed.
6. When the juice stops flowing, remove the pitcher, add the cinnamon, and stir the juice.
7. Serve immediately.

VARIATION TIP: Other spices known to reduce inflammation include ginger, turmeric, clove, rosemary, cayenne pepper, cumin, and sage. Try just a pinch of one of these other spices in place of the cinnamon in this recipe.

PER SERVING: CALORIES: 106; TOTAL FAT: 1G; SUGAR: 20G; CARBOHYDRATES: 33G; FIBER: 1G; PROTEIN: 3G

SIMPLE DETOX JUICE

Makes 1 (16-ounce) serving **Prep time:** 15 minutes

If detox is your goal, cilantro is your herb. Cilantro binds with toxins in your body, then flushes them out. Lemons help balance your pH, while celery and cucumbers keep you hydrated.

1 cucumber
1 bunch cilantro
5 celery ribs
2 lemons

1. Wash all the ingredients.
2. Trim the ends from the cucumber and celery, then cut into 4-inch pieces.
3. Peel the lemons and cut into quarters.
4. Place a pitcher under the juicer's spout to collect the juice.
5. Feed each ingredient through the juicer's intake tube in the order listed.
6. When the juice stops flowing, remove the pitcher and stir the juice.
7. Serve immediately.

HEALTH TIP: Another simple morning drink is warm lemon water. One cup of warm water plus a slice of lemon increases your metabolic rate, promotes digestion and weight loss, and reduces inflammation.

PER SERVING: CALORIES: 77; TOTAL FAT: 1G; SUGAR: 10G; CARBOHYDRATES: 28G; FIBER: 1G; PROTEIN: 5G

GREENS 'N' GARLIC

Makes 1 (12-ounce) serving **Prep time:** 15 minutes

Do you feel like you're coming down with a cold? The garlic in this juice will help fight those germs, and the leafy greens will boost your immune system and give you the power to handle most anything.

1½ cucumbers
2 cups spinach
½ cup green cabbage
3 carrots
1 garlic clove, peeled
1 lemon

1. Wash all the ingredients except the garlic.
2. Trim the ends from the cucumbers and carrots, then cut into 4-inch pieces.
3. Cut the cabbage in half, then slice or chop into smaller pieces.
4. Peel the lemon and cut into quarters.
5. Place a pitcher under the juicer's spout to collect the juice.
6. Feed each ingredient through the juicer's intake tube in the order listed.
7. When the juice stops flowing, remove the pitcher and stir the juice.
8. Serve immediately.

DID YOU KNOW? Research shows that raw garlic is even better for your body than cooked garlic, which loses some vitamins and minerals in the heating process.

PER SERVING: CALORIES: 121; TOTAL FAT: 1G; SUGAR: 16G; CARBOHYDRATES: 41G; FIBER: 2G; PROTEIN: 6G

CLEANSE ASSIST

Makes 1 (12-ounce) serving **Prep time:** 15 minutes

Dandelion greens are not just a pesky weed. Dandelion is also a valuable herb. This bitter plant tones, detoxifies, and helps ease joint pain, eczema, and PMS. The dandelion in this healthy juice is perfectly palatable.

---

2 cups kale
½ cup dandelion
greens 1 pear
½ lemon

1. Wash all the ingredients.
2. Cut the pear into quarters, removing the core and seeds, but leaving the peel intact.
3. Peel the lemon half and cut into quarters.
4. Place a pitcher under the juicer's spout to collect the juice.
5. Feed each ingredient through the juicer's intake tube in the order listed.
6. When the juice stops flowing, remove the pitcher and stir the juice.
7. Serve immediately.

INGREDIENT TIP: Tea made from dandelion greens is a popular drink to help stimulate mucus production and detoxification. Cut dandelion leaves into small pieces and add 1 teaspoon to 1 cup of nearly boiling water. Let steep for 5 minutes.

PER SERVING: CALORIES: 162; TOTAL FAT: 2G; SUGAR: 22G; CARBOHYDRATES: 50G; FIBER: 2G; PROTEIN: 10G

GINGER BLAST

Makes 1 (12-ounce) serving **Prep time:** 15 minutes

This homemade version of ginger ale is a great stomach tonic and a refreshing drink for any occasion. Spinach gives an extra immune boost, and cherries are great for reducing inflammation, especially if you suffer from arthritis.

1½ cups spinach
1 cup cherries
Fresh ginger root
1 cup sparkling water

1. Wash the spinach, cherries, and ginger root.
2. Remove the cherry pits and stems.
3. Slice off a 2-inch piece of the ginger root.
4. Place a pitcher under the juicer's spout to collect the juice.
5. Feed each ingredient through the juicer's intake tube in the order listed.
6. When the juice stops flowing, remove the pitcher and stir the juice.
7. Serve immediately.

INGREDIENT TIP: True sparkling water contains minerals and is obtained from an underground source. The water takes in minerals from the layers of natural rock it flows through. I recommend buying sparkling water brands that contain minerals instead of added flavors.

PER SERVING: CALORIES: 76; TOTAL FAT: 0G; SUGAR: 14G; CARBOHYDRATES: 21G; FIBER: 1G; PROTEIN: 2G

IMMUNITY PLUS

Makes 1 (12-ounce) serving **Prep time:** 15 minutes

When your immune system is strong, your body can more easily fight off viral infections and chronic ailments. Antioxidants like vitamin C are key factors in building your immune system, and this juice has it in spades.

---

1 small beet
2 carrots
8 celery ribs
1 broccoli stalk
2 garlic cloves, peeled

1. Wash all the ingredients except the garlic.
2. Remove any greens from the beet and save for juicing later. Cut the beet into quarters.
3. Trim the ends from the carrots and celery, then cut into 4-inch pieces.
4. Remove the stalk from the broccoli crown with a knife and discard or save to juice later. Cut the crown into small florets.
5. Place a pitcher under the juicer's spout to collect the juice.
6. Feed each ingredient through the juicer's intake tube in the order listed.
7. When the juice stops flowing, remove the pitcher and stir the juice.
8. Serve immediately.

DID YOU KNOW? Some people experience changes in their bowel movements after consuming beets or beet juice. Don't be alarmed by a red tinge in the stool.

PER SERVING: CALORIES: 120; TOTAL FAT: 1G; SUGAR: 17G; CARBOHYDRATES: 34G; FIBER: 2G; PROTEIN: 7G

ALOE CLEANSER

Makes 1 (8-ounce) serving **Prep time:** 10 minutes

Aloe vera juice may improve digestion and reduce the incidence of stomach ulcers. When combined with alfalfa sprouts, aloe vera juice can help reduce the risk of breast cancer, prevent osteoporosis, and brighten skin.

¼ cup alfalfa sprouts
1 pear
1 cup cabbage
¼ cup aloe vera juice

1. Wash the alfalfa sprouts, pear, and cabbage.
2. Cut the pear into quarters, removing the core and seeds, but leaving the peel intact.
3. Cut the cabbage in half, then slice or chop into smaller pieces.
4. Place a pitcher under the juicer's spout to collect the juice.
5. Feed the first three ingredients through the juicer's intake tube in the order listed.
6. When the juice stops flowing, remove the pitcher, add the aloe vera juice, and stir.
7. Serve immediately.

HEALTH TIP: Aloe vera juice can be used externally as a skin-care tonic to remove dirt and impurities. It also can provide relief from minor burns and insect bites.

PER SERVING: CALORIES: 91; TOTAL FAT: 0G; SUGAR: 17G; CARBOHYDRATES: 29G; FIBER: 1G; PROTEIN: 3G

GOOD, GOOD, GOOD DIGESTION

Makes 1 (12-ounce) serving **Prep time:** 15 minutes

Good digestion is critical to your overall health. Some people believe disease originates in the gut, so when you treat your digestive tract well, you're treating your entire body well. Papaya contains wonderful enzymes that do the trick when it comes to digestion.

---

1 cup papaya
6 kale leaves
Fresh turmeric root
1 lemon

1. Wash the kale, turmeric root, and lemon.
2. Cut the papaya in half lengthwise. Scoop out seeds and discard, then scoop out flesh and discard the papaya skin.
3. Slice off a 2-inch piece of the turmeric root.
4. Peel the lemon and cut into quarters.
5. Place a pitcher under the juicer's spout to collect the juice.
6. Feed each ingredient through the juicer's intake tube in the order listed.
7. When the juice stops flowing, remove the pitcher, and stir the juice.
8. Serve immediately.

DID YOU KNOW? Papain, the main enzyme in papaya, aids digestion by breaking proteins down into smaller fragments and by allowing greater absorption of vitamins and minerals.

PER SERVING: CALORIES: 127; TOTAL FAT: 2G; SUGAR: 14G; CARBOHYDRATES: 36G; FIBER: 1G; PROTEIN: 8G

VITAMIN C CELEBRATION

Makes 1 (8-ounce) serving **Prep time:** 15 minutes

Vitamin C is needed by every part of your body to grow and repair tissues. When consumed regularly, vitamin C helps build your immune system so viral colds stay away. You'll want to drink this juice often for its citrusy, sweet flavor.

---

1 orange
½ red bell pepper
1 cup broccoli
2 collard green
leaves ¼ cucumber

1. Wash all the ingredients.
2. Peel the orange and cut into quarters.
3. Remove the stem and seeds from the bell pepper. Cut into small pieces.
4. Remove the stalk from the broccoli crown with a knife and discard or save to juice later. Cut the crown into small florets.
5. Trim the ends from the cucumber, then cut into quarters.
6. Place a pitcher under the juicer's spout to collect the juice.
7. Feed each ingredient through the juicer's intake tube in the order listed.
8. When the juice stops flowing, remove the pitcher and stir the juice.
9. Serve immediately.

DID YOU KNOW? Red bell peppers are actually green bell peppers that have remained on the plant to ripen. The red ones contain twice the vitamin C content of green bell peppers and taste sweeter, which makes them more popular for juicing and eating raw.

PER SERVING: CALORIES: 81; TOTAL FAT: 1G; SUGAR: 15G; CARBOHYDRATES: 24G;

FIBER: 1G; PROTEIN: 4G

HEALTHY HEALING GREENS

Makes 1 (10-ounce) serving **Prep time:** 15 minutes

There's no fruit in this green juice, but you won't miss it at all. This recipe calls for mild and relatively sweet veggies that also boast great healing properties for your eyes, skin, heart, and immune system. The taste of this juice is mostly sweet, slightly salty, and earthy.

---

2 cups spinach
3 cups broccoli
4 celery ribs
2 carrots

1. Wash all the ingredients.
2. Remove the stalk from the broccoli crown with a knife and discard or save to juice later. Cut the crown into small florets.
3. Trim the ends from the celery and carrots, then cut into 4-inch pieces.
4. Place a pitcher under the juicer's spout to collect the juice.
5. Feed each ingredient through the juicer's intake tube in the order listed.
6. When the juice stops flowing, remove the pitcher and stir the juice.
7. Serve immediately.

DID YOU KNOW? Baby carrots have the same amount of sugar as regular carrots but less iron, phosphorus, and magnesium. They also contain less vitamin A and C but more folate.

PER SERVING: CALORIES: 69; TOTAL FAT: 1G; SUGAR: 7G; CARBOHYDRATES: 20G; FIBER: 1G; PROTEIN: 6G

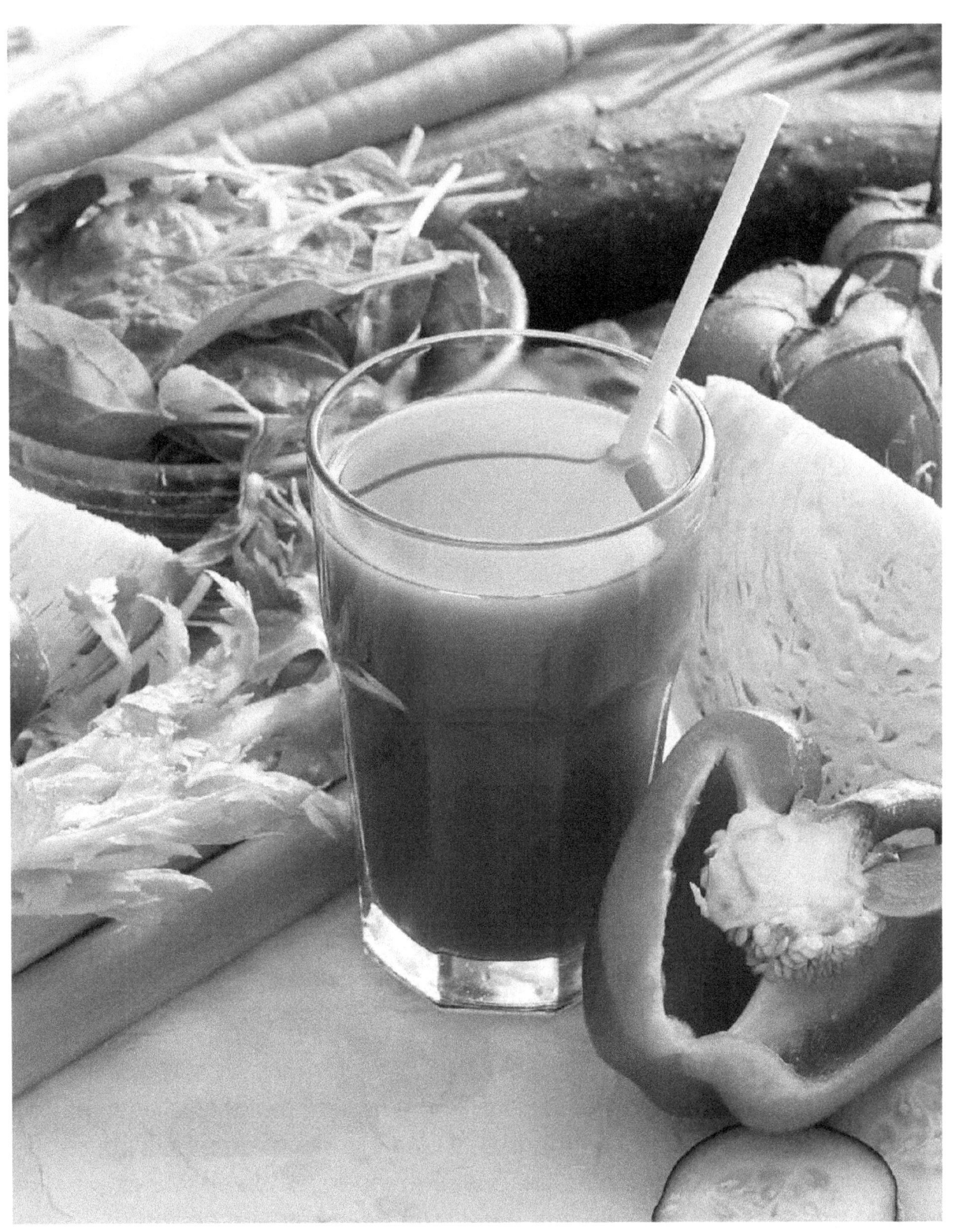

VEGETABLE 8

8
Your Daily Dose of Green

Beta-Carotene Greens

Alkalizing Greens

Vegetable 8

Salad in a Glass

Green Turbo

Veggies 'n' Sprouts

Kitchen Sink Green Juice

Slice of Life

Live Well Green Juice

Chlorophyll Boost

Epic Green Juice

I Dream of Green

Now and Zen Green Juice

Emerald Alkalizing Juice

The Daily Fix

While you may be accustomed to eating three meals a day, nutrition experts encourage us to consider other routines for getting the fuel we need. Some experts advise intermittent fasting, which is eating during very limited hours. Others advise eating many smaller meals throughout the day. My advice is to find a routine that works best for you. One thing is certain, though: Consuming lots of greens is ideal. The recipes in this chapter offer a well-rounded supply of vitamins and minerals that will help you meet your daily nutrition goals.

BETA-CAROTENE GREENS

Makes 1 (12-ounce) serving **Prep time:** 15 minutes

Carrots and dark, leafy greens are high in beta-carotene, which the body converts into vitamin A. Your skin, mucous membranes, immune system, and vision require this vitamin for optimal health. Drink this rich juice to give you energy and stamina all day.

- 4 Swiss chard leaves
- 4 kale leaves
- 4 carrots
- 1 green bell pepper
- 1 lemon

1. Wash all the ingredients.
2. Trim the ends from the carrots, then cut into 4-inch pieces.
3. Remove the stem and seeds from the bell pepper. Cut into small pieces.
4. Peel the lemon and cut into quarters.
5. Place a pitcher under the juicer's spout to collect the juice.
6. Feed each ingredient through the juicer's intake tube in the order listed.
7. When the juice stops flowing, remove the pitcher and stir the juice.
8. Serve immediately.

DID YOU KNOW? Eating carrots may help improve eyesight in low-light conditions, research shows. Carrots contain beta-carotene, a pigment that nourishes the eye and helps the body make vitamin A. Vitamin A, in turn, allows the eye to transmit light as a signal to the brain, allowing people to see under lowlight conditions.

PER SERVING: CALORIES: 130; TOTAL FAT: 2G; SUGAR: 15G; CARBOHYDRATES: 40G; FIBER: 2G; PROTEIN: 10G

ALKALIZING GREENS

Makes 1 (12-ounce) serving **Prep time:** 15 minutes

Your body seeks homeostasis, or balance. A body that measures more alkaline tends to be healthier and gets sick less often. Alkalinity is measured chemically on a pH scale (from 0 to 14). Processed foods lower alkalinity and make your body more acidic.

---

2 cups spinach
1 cucumber
1 cup broccoli
2 kale leaves
1 green apple
1 lemon

1. Wash all the ingredients.
2. Remove the stalk from the broccoli crown with a knife and discard or save to juice later. Cut the crown into small florets.
3. Remove the apple core and discard. Cut the apple into quarters, leaving the peel intact.
4. Peel the lemon and cut into quarters.
5. Place a pitcher under the juicer's spout to collect the juice.
6. Feed each ingredient through the juicer's intake tube in the order listed.
7. When the juice stops flowing, remove the pitcher and stir the juice.
8. Serve immediately.

HEALTH TIP: Regular aerobic exercise, such as a brisk walk, restores the pH balance in your body by increasing your metabolism.

PER SERVING: CALORIES: 122; TOTAL FAT: 1G; SUGAR: 18G; CARBOHYDRATES: 38G; FIBER: 1G; PROTEIN: 7G

VEGETABLE 8

Makes 1 (12-ounce) serving **Prep time:** 20 minutes

This healthier version of the classic store-bought juice contains no additives and provides you with an array of vitamins and minerals. Vitamin A boosts your immune system, while vitamin C assists with bone health and injury repair. Potassium helps regulate blood pressure and muscle growth. Robust in flavor and texture, this drink will fill you up and keep you going for hours.

---

2 medium tomatoes
1 cucumber
1 cup spinach
1 cup cabbage
½ red bell pepper
2 celery ribs
2 carrots
1 green onion

1. Wash all the ingredients.
2. Remove stems from the tomatoes and cut into quarters.
3. Trim the ends from the cucumber, celery, carrots, and green onion, then cut into 4-inch pieces.
4. Cut cabbage in half, then slice or chop into smaller pieces.
5. Remove the stem and seeds from the bell pepper. Cut into small pieces.
6. Place a pitcher under the juicer's spout to collect the juice.
7. Feed each ingredient through the juicer's intake tube in the order listed.
8. When the juice stops flowing, remove the pitcher and stir the juice.
9. Serve immediately.

DID YOU KNOW? How many vegetables does it take to make 1 cup of juice? One English cucumber will yield 1 cup of juice, as will 9 medium carrots, 1 bunch of celery, or 3 medium tomatoes.

PER SERVING: CALORIES: 104; TOTAL FAT: 1G; SUGAR: 16G; CARBOHYDRATES: 30G; FIBER: 1G; PROTEIN: 6G

SALAD IN A GLASS

Makes 1 (12-ounce) serving **Prep time:** 15 minutes

What would you get if you made a salad, then put all the ingredients through your juicer? This juice! An on-the-go meal for busy people, this juice is bursting with greens for healthy blood and tomatoes and peppers to support your eyes. It also contains carrots for glowing skin and parsley to trap toxins lurking in your body.

---

3 carrots
6 romaine lettuce leaves
2 medium tomatoes
2 green onions
½ green bell pepper
¼ cup parsley
½ lemon

1. Wash all the ingredients.
2. Trim the ends from carrots and green onions, then cut into 4-inch pieces.
3. Remove the stems from the tomatoes and cut into quarters.
4. Remove the stem and seeds from the bell pepper. Cut into small pieces.
5. Peel the lemon half and cut into quarters.
6. Place a pitcher under the juicer's spout to collect the juice.
7. Feed each ingredient through the juicer's intake tube in the order listed.
8. When the juice stops flowing, remove the pitcher and stir the juice.
9. Serve immediately.

VARIATION TIP: For a lighter, less sweet version of this juice, substitute zucchini or yellow squash for the carrots.

PER SERVING: CALORIES: 89; TOTAL FAT: 1G; SUGAR: 14G; CARBOHYDRATES: 28G; FIBER: 1G; PROTEIN: 5G

GREEN TURBO

Makes 1 (12-ounce) serving **Prep time:** 15 minutes

As they say, you are what you eat or, in this case, drink. The greens in this recipe offer a full variety of nutrients from vitamins A, C, K, and B to protein and potassium. After drinking this juice, you will feel supercharged, like a turbo engine, raring to go.

½ cup spinach
3 kale leaves
2 green apples
2 celery ribs
½ cup parsley
1 cucumber
½ lemon
Fresh ginger root

1. Wash all the ingredients.
2. Remove the apple core and discard. Cut the apples into quarters, leaving the peel intact.
3. Trim the ends from the celery and cucumber, then cut into 4-inch pieces.
4. Peel the lemon half and cut into quarters.
5. Slice off a ½-inch piece of fresh ginger root.
6. Place a pitcher under the juicer's spout to collect the juice.
7. Feed each ingredient through the juicer's intake tube in the order listed.
8. When the juice stops flowing, remove the pitcher and stir the juice.
9. Serve immediately.

INGREDIENT TIP: Parsley kills odor-producing bacteria that results in bad breath and possible tooth enamel loss. Chew parsley leaves after meals to help freshen your breath.

PER SERVING: CALORIES: 173; TOTAL FAT: 2G; SUGAR: 29G; CARBOHYDRATES: 53G; FIBER: 2G; PROTEIN: 7G

VEGGIES 'N' SPROUTS

Makes 1 (12-ounce) serving **Prep time:** 10 minutes

The vitamins and minerals in alfalfa sprouts are alkaline and easy for the body to absorb and use to protect against diseases like cancer. Alfalfa sprouts have a mild and nutty flavor, and they are best eaten raw in salads, on sandwiches, and in juices like this one.

---

4 celery ribs
1 cucumber
8 lettuce leaves
½ cup alfalfa sprouts

1. Wash all the ingredients.
2. Trim the ends from the celery and cucumber, then cut into 4-inch pieces.
3. Place a pitcher under the juicer's spout to collect the juice.
4. Feed each ingredient through the juicer's intake tube in the order listed.
5. When the juice stops flowing, remove the pitcher and stir the juice.
6. Serve immediately.

VARIATION TIP: Alfalfa sprouts are easy to find in the grocery store, but feel free to substitute broccoli sprouts or clover sprouts in this juice.

PER SERVING: CALORIES: 55; TOTAL FAT: 1G; SUGAR: 7G; CARBOHYDRATES: 16G; FIBER: 1G; PROTEIN: 5G

KITCHEN SINK GREEN JUICE

Makes 1 (12-ounce) serving **Prep time:** 15 minutes

As a kid, I picked beans from the garden and put them into a sink full of water to wash and snap. I still love doing that today, only I buy the beans from the local farmers market whenever I can. Enjoy this bright, mild green juice any time of year and especially in May through September when green beans are in peak season.

1 cup spinach
2 cups green beans
1 cucumber
½ pear
½ lemon

1. Wash all the ingredients.
2. Trim the ends from the green beans and cucumber, then cut into 4-inch pieces.
3. Cut the pear into quarters, removing the core and seeds, but leaving the peel intact.
4. Peel the lemon half and cut into quarters.
5. Place a pitcher under the juicer's spout to collect the juice.
6. Feed each ingredient through the juicer's intake tube in the order listed.
7. When the juice stops flowing, remove the pitcher and stir the juice.
8. Serve immediately.

VARIATION TIP: Don't have all the ingredients in your kitchen? Try one or more of these substitutions:

spinach—basil
green beans—zucchini

cucumber—celery
pear—apple
lemon—lime

PER SERVING: CALORIES: 102; TOTAL FAT: 1G; SUGAR: 16G; CARBOHYDRATES: 34G; FIBER: 1G; PROTEIN: 6G

SLICE OF LIFE

Makes 1 (10-ounce) serving **Prep time:** 15 minutes

Summertime is melon time, especially in my family. We love to sit outside with slices of watermelon in hand, ready to spit seeds and have a good laugh. My grandfather used to say that salt made the watermelon taste sweeter. To honor him, I've added some celery to this refreshing drink.

1½ cups watermelon
4 kale leaves
½ lime
2 celery ribs

1. Wash the kale, lime, and celery.
2. Cut the watermelon into quarters. Remove the rind and discard. Cut the watermelon into smaller pieces.
3. Trim the ends from the celery, then cut into 4-inch pieces.
4. Peel the lime half and cut into quarters.
5. Place a pitcher under the juicer's spout to collect the juice.
6. Feed each ingredient through the juicer's intake tube in the order listed.
7. When the juice stops flowing, remove the pitcher and stir the juice.
8. Serve immediately.

VARIATION TIP: Summertime is also popsicle weather. Pour this juice into some popsicle molds for a sweet frozen treat.

PER SERVING: CALORIES: 90; TOTAL FAT: 1G; SUGAR: 13G; CARBOHYDRATES: 24G; FIBER: 1G; PROTEIN: 6G

LIVE WELL GREEN JUICE

Makes 1 (12-ounce) serving **Prep time:** 15 minutes

Watercress is a cruciferous green that is often said to be the most nutrient-dense vegetable. It has a peppery taste, and its benefits include supporting bone health and reducing cancer risk.

---

2 cups spinach
1 cup clover sprouts
1 cup watercress
2 green apples
2 cups broccoli

1. Wash all the ingredients.
2. Remove the apple cores and discard. Cut the apples into quarters, leaving the peel intact.
3. Remove the stalk from the broccoli crown with a knife and discard or save to juice later. Cut the crown into small florets.
4. Place a pitcher under the juicer's spout to collect the juice.
5. Feed each ingredient through the juicer's intake tube in the order listed.
6. When the juice stops flowing, remove the pitcher and stir the juice.
7. Serve immediately.

DID YOU KNOW? Watercress is native to Europe and Asia. It grows in shallow, moving water and resembles a green mat or carpet.

PER SERVING: CALORIES: 114; TOTAL FAT: 1G; SUGAR: 23G; CARBOHYDRATES: 34G; FIBER: 1G; PROTEIN: 5G

CHLOROPHYLL BOOST

Makes 1 (12-ounce) serving **Prep time:** 15 minutes

Drink this green juice to feel like you're on a tropical island paradise. The flavor is dense and briny, like you might imagine the ocean to taste. Spirulina, a superfood, supports heart and gut health and boosts metabolism. One study suggests that with regular consumption, spirulina reduces body mass index.

---

1 cup pineapple
4 kale leaves
1 cup spinach
½ cucumber 7
mint leaves
½ teaspoon spirulina powder

1. Wash the kale, spinach, cucumber, and mint.
2. Trim the ends and skin from the pineapple, then remove core and discard. Cut pineapple into 1-inch chunks.
3. Trim the ends from the cucumber, then cut into 4-inch pieces.
4. Place a pitcher under the juicer's spout to collect the juice.
5. Feed the first five ingredients through the juicer's intake tube in the order listed.
6. When the juice stops flowing, remove the pitcher, add the spirulina powder, and stir.
7. Serve immediately.

INGREDIENT TIP: When used in a facial steam, mint leaves can help clear your sinuses. Bring a pot of water to boil, add a few mint leaves, and turn off the heat. Drape a towel over your head and carefully lean over the pot to breathe in the fresh scent.

PER SERVING: CALORIES: 103; TOTAL FAT: 1G; SUGAR: 15G; CARBOHYDRATES: 28G; FIBER: 1G; PROTEIN: 6G

EPIC GREEN JUICE

Makes 1 (12-ounce) serving **Prep time:** 15 minutes

Turnips are loaded with vitamins C and B6 and contribute to bowel regularity, a healthy heart, weight loss, and cancer prevention. Turnips taste similar to radishes or rutabagas, slightly peppery and bitter, but the sweetness of the pear and cantaloupe in this recipe makes for a smooth, sweeter finish.

---

1 turnip with greens
1 pear
1 cup spinach
½ cucumber
1 cup cantaloupe

1. Wash the turnip, pear, spinach, and cucumber.
2. Trim the greens and cut the turnip into small chunks.
3. Cut the pear into quarters, removing the core and seeds, but leaving the peel intact.
4. Trim the ends from the cucumber, then cut into 4-inch pieces.
5. Cut the cantaloupe into quarters. Remove the rind, scoop out the seeds, and discard. Cut the cantaloupe into small pieces.
6. Place a pitcher under the juicer's spout to collect the juice.
7. Feed each ingredient through the juicer's intake tube in the order listed.
8. When the juice stops flowing, remove the pitcher and stir the juice.
9. Serve immediately.

INGREDIENT TIP: Use your nose when choosing a cantaloupe. This fruit should have a sweet, slightly musky scent. The cantaloupe should feel relatively heavy in relation to its size and have a stem end that gives slightly when you press it with your thumb.

PER SERVING: CALORIES: 133; TOTAL FAT: 1G; SUGAR: 26G; CARBOHYDRATES: 40G; FIBER: 1G; PROTEIN: 4G

I DREAM OF GREEN

Makes 1 (10-ounce) serving **Prep time:** 15 minutes

Don't be surprised if you wake up in the morning craving this juice. It's a delicious blend of honeydew melon and greens. Honeydew is rich in folate, vitamin K, and magnesium, all of which support healthy bones.

1 cup honeydew melon
4 collard green leaves
3 cups cabbage
1 lemon

1. Wash the collard greens, cabbage, and lemon.
2. Cut the honeydew melon into quarters. Remove the rind and discard. Cut the melon into small pieces.
3. Cut the cabbage in half, then slice or chop into smaller pieces.
4. Peel the lemon and cut into quarters.
5. Place a pitcher under the juicer's spout to collect the juice.
6. Feed each ingredient through the juicer's intake tube in the order listed.
7. When the juice stops flowing, remove the pitcher and stir the juice.
8. Serve immediately.

INGREDIENT TIP: Honeydew melon seeds make a great snack. Rinse them and pat them dry. Toss the seeds with olive oil and salt, then spread them on a baking sheet and roast in a 325°F oven for 20 to 40 minutes.

PER SERVING: CALORIES: 85; TOTAL FAT: 1G; SUGAR: 16G; CARBOHYDRATES: 29G; FIBER: 1G; PROTEIN: 5G

NOW AND ZEN GREEN JUICE

Makes 1 (8-ounce) serving **Prep time:** 15 minutes

The Zen way is to learn through experience in the moment. For instance, how can you know if you like asparagus juice until you've tried it? Well, here is your opportunity. Make a glass of this relaxing juice and sip away.

2 kiwis
6 asparagus spears
4 celery ribs
4 kale leaves

1. Wash all the ingredients.
2. Peel the kiwis, then cut them into quarters. (There's no need to peel them unless you want to.)
3. Trim the bottoms of the asparagus, then cut into small pieces.
4. Trim the ends from the celery, then cut into 4-inch pieces.
5. Place a pitcher under the juicer's spout to collect the juice.
6. Feed each ingredient through the juicer's intake tube in the order listed.
7. When the juice stops flowing, remove the pitcher and stir the juice.
8. Serve immediately.

INGREDIENT TIP: You can use excess raw asparagus spears to make a delicious salad. Shave the spears with a vegetable peeler, then add lemon juice, olive oil, and parmesan cheese (if desired).

PER SERVING: CALORIES: 108; TOTAL FAT: 2G; SUGAR: 14G; CARBOHYDRATES: 30G; FIBER: 2G; PROTEIN: 8G

EMERALD ALKALIZING JUICE

Makes 1 (10-ounce) serving **Prep time:** 15 minutes

This juice combines spinach for strength, wheatgrass for energy, and apple cider vinegar to raise your pH and boost your immune system. The chlorophyll content of spinach and wheatgrass gives this juice its rich green color. The spinach and wheatgrass, along with apple cider vinegar, work together to help your body absorb nutrients, rebuild tissues, reduce inflammation, and strengthen the blood.

---

3 cups spinach
1 red apple
½ cucumber
¼ cup filtered water
½ tablespoon wheatgrass powder
1 tablespoon apple cider vinegar

1. Wash the spinach, apple, and cucumber.
2. Remove the apple core and discard. Cut the apple into quarters, leaving the peel intact.
3. Trim the ends from the cucumber, then cut into 4-inch pieces.
4. Place a pitcher under the juicer's spout to collect the juice.
5. Feed the first three ingredients through the juicer's intake tube in the order listed.
6. When the juice stops flowing, remove the pitcher, add the water, wheatgrass powder and apple cider vinegar, and stir the juice.
7. Serve immediately.

DID YOU KNOW? There are approximately one hundred cucumber varieties. The three most popular are pickling, slicing, and English cucumbers. Any of these are great for juicing.

PER SERVING: CALORIES: 98; TOTAL FAT: 1G; SUGAR: 13G; CARBOHYDRATES: 22G; FIBER: 2G; PROTEIN: 5G

THE DAILY FIX

Makes 1 (8-ounce) serving **Prep time:** 10 minutes

There are some days when you need an extra boost of protein, and you want to get your greens in without juicing any fruits. This recipe is your answer. Coconut water boasts a nutty, fresh flavor, and when you add your favorite protein powder to the mix, you'll wonder how you ever got along before this delicious and nutritious juice.

---

1 cup mixed greens
½ cucumber
½ cup coconut water
1 scoop protein powder

1. Wash the greens and cucumber.
2. Trim the ends from the cucumber, then cut into 4-inch pieces.
3. Place a pitcher under the juicer's spout to collect the juice.
4. Feed the first two ingredients through the juicer's intake tube in the order listed.
5. When the juice stops flowing, remove the pitcher, add the coconut water and protein powder, and stir.
6. Serve immediately.

INGREDIENT TIP: Unopened coconut water will last up to a year on a cool, dark shelf. After opening your coconut water, seal it in an airtight container and store it in the refrigerator for up to 3 days.

PER SERVING: CALORIES: 169; TOTAL FAT: 2G; SUGAR: 4G; CARBOHYDRATES: 19G; FIBER: 0G; PROTEIN: 22G

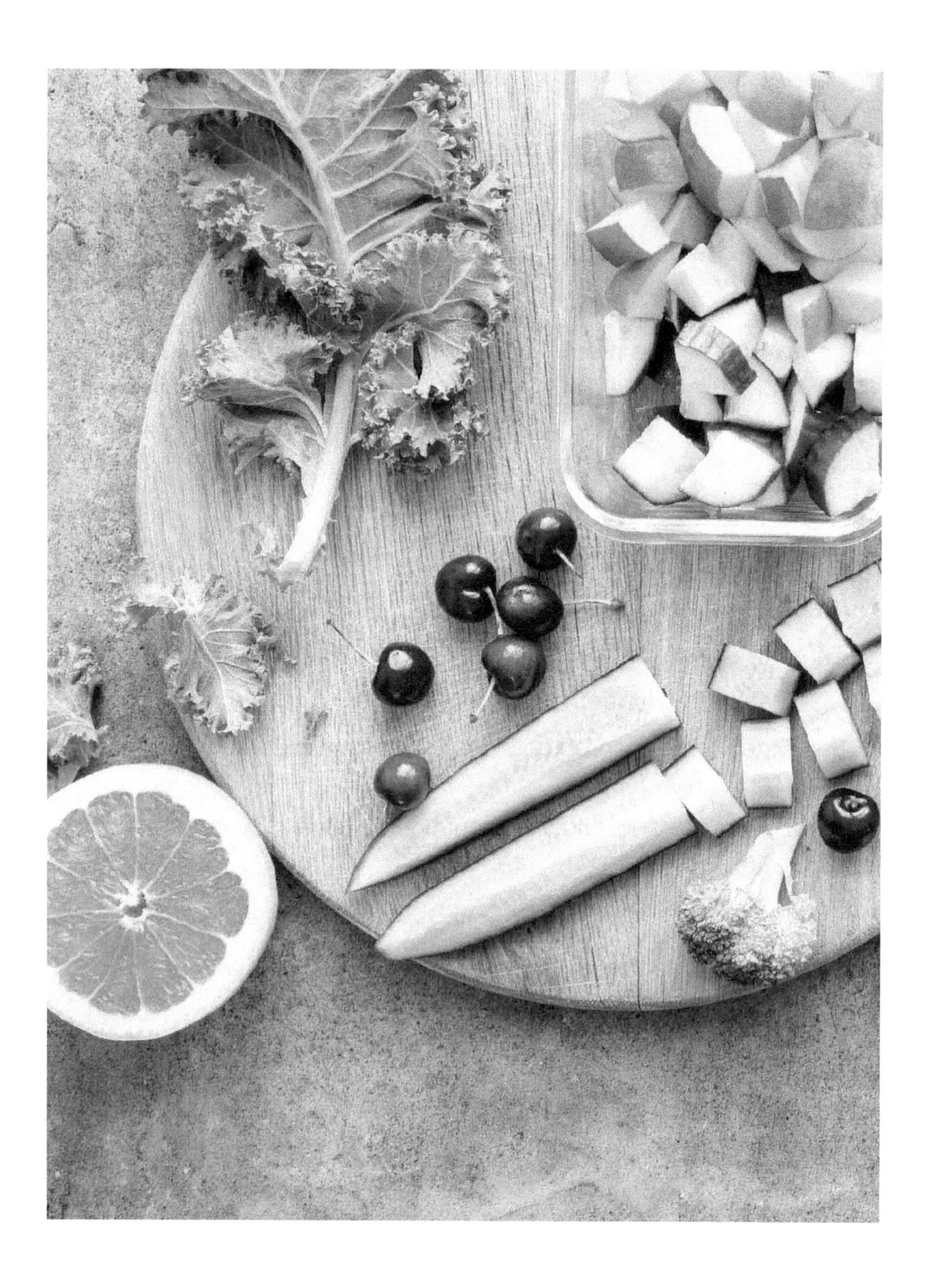

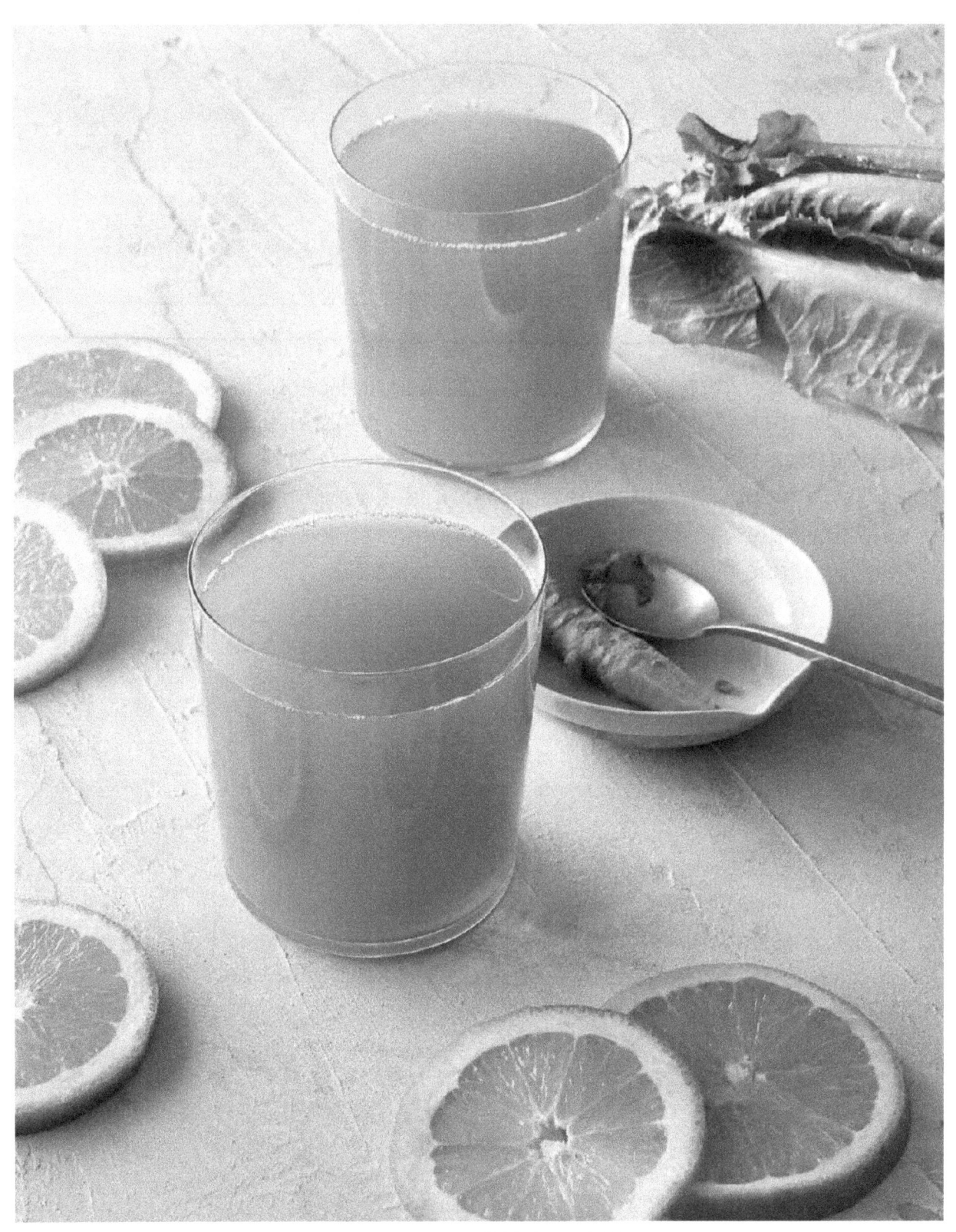

HAPPY FACE GREEN JUICE

9

The Three-Day Green Cleanse

Sometimes I still feel sluggish despite my best efforts to live a healthy life. When this happens, I practice self-care in the form of a juice cleanse. A juice cleanse is when you consume only water and juices (no solid food) for a short period of time, typically three days. In that time, the body expends most of its energy removing waste and pollutants, allowing you to feel lighter and more energized. A juice cleanse essentially resets the body so everything functions better. You can expect to have an improved sense of taste, less cravings for junk food, clearer skin, more efficient bowel movements, and even a small amount of weight loss.

WHO SHOULD CLEANSE?

Generally, a juice cleanse is a safe method of maintaining good health. However, it is not advised for people with certain conditions such as:
- An extremely weakened immune system
- Diabetes
- Anemia
- Pregnant or nursing
- Children under 18
- Anorexia, bulimia, or malnutrition
- Heart failure
- Liver failure
- Kidney failure
- Tuberculosis
- Low blood pressure

Because the body is composed of a complex set of systems, we are not always aware of our true state of health. Please consult with a qualified health practitioner to assess your health before beginning any new health routine like a juice cleanse.

WHEN TO CLEANSE

It's safe to do a short juice cleanse up to four times per year. In order to determine when you should cleanse, you will need to pay attention to how your body feels and functions. Several indicators of a body out of balance include cravings for junk food, feeling bloated, constipation, difficulty thinking clearly, low energy, and breakouts or unusually dry skin.

Pick a time to start your cleanse when you predict the lowest amount of stress, such as the weekend. Cleansing works best when you can detach from the outside world and focus on you.

BEFORE THE CLEANSE

It can be tempting to start a cleanse the moment you've decided to do it, however, it's important to plan and prepare your body before you begin. Your body will respond better if you take a few days to transition into a juice cleanse, especially if you are not accustomed to eating a primarily vegetarian diet.

Three to seven days before your cleanse incorporate the following into your diet:

- Eat more fruits and vegetables
- Cut back or eliminate red meats, cheeses, packaged foods, and refined sugars
- Eat fiber-rich foods or take a fiber supplement to move the bowels
- Drink at least eight glasses of water per day to help flush toxins
- Substitute herbal tea for coffee in the morning as coffee can dehydrate the body, making the liver work harder
- Avoid alcohol as it affects the liver, one of the main detoxification organs

DURING THE CLEANSE

Your routine during a juice cleanse will likely be very different than your regular daily routine. For three consecutive days you will consume six juices per day, throughout the day, each consisting of 10 to 16 ounces of liquid. You will not eat any solid foods during this cleanse. As your body and mind adapt to this change, you may feel some highs and lows.

Follow these five guidelines to stay focused and successful during your juice cleanse.

1. If you feel hungry, make another juice or drink a glass of water. Try occupying your mind with an activity to distract from your hunger for the time being. If after attempting both hunger strategies, you still feel the urge to eat something, peel a cucumber, slice it and then eat one slice, chewing slowly. Observe how your body feels after doing

this.

2. Movement is important during a juice cleanse. Your mind and body will welcome light exercise. Walking or stretching are your best options. However, avoid heavy lifting or high-intensity exercises. You can resume regular exercise after your cleanse is complete.

3. As your body begins to detoxify, you may find that you are more tired than usual at the end of the day. Proper rest each night, at least seven to eight hours, will ensure the body can do what it needs to do to recover. An added benefit is that you will wake up feeling refreshed both mentally and physically.

4. You will be drinking three different juices each day. Make your juice for each day the evening before so you have no worries or temptations in the morning to quit the cleanse.

5. Much of the challenge of a juice cleanse is mental. You may be tempted to eat solid food based on your environment. Try to limit situations that may create such temptations. For example, avoid restaurants and food programs on television. If you must prepare food for your family, ask someone to help you in the kitchen.

THE THREE-DAY GREEN CLEANSE

This three-day cleanse was designed to be simple yet effective. The juices have been chosen for their variety of ingredients, nutrition, and ease of preparation. You may choice to make substitutions if desired, for instance swapping out spinach for kale, or choose your own juices from the recipes in this book if you feel confident in doing so. Always pay attention to how your body feels. Slight headaches and discomfort or aches in your body are to be expected, however nausea and vomiting are not. If these latter symptoms arise, discontinue the cleanse. And in addition to a glass of lemon water upon rising, remember to continue drinking water throughout the day.

The Three-Day Juicing Cleanse: DAY 1

After waking up drink 1 (8-ounce) glass of water with the juice of ½ lemon

8:00 a.m.: Green Hydrating Juice

10:30 a.m.: Green Hydrating Juice

12:00 p.m.: Happy Face Green Juice

3:00 p.m.: Happy Face Green Juice

6:00 p.m.: Grapes and Greens

8:30 p.m.: Grapes and Greens

The Three-Day Juicing Cleanse: DAY 2

After waking up drink 1 (8-ounce) glass of water with the juice of ½ lemon

8:00 a.m.:	Sunrise Special
10:30 a.m.:	Sunrise Special
12:00 p.m.:	Make My Day Juice
3:00 p.m.:	Make My Day Juice
6:00 p.m.:	Electrolyte Power Juice
8:30 p.m.:	Electrolyte Power Juice

The Three-Day Juicing Cleanse: DAY 3

After waking up drink 1 (8 ounce) glass of water with juice of ½ lemon

8:00 a.m.:	Alkalizing Greens
10:30 a.m.:	Alkalizing Greens

12:00 p.m.: Make My Day Juice

3:00 p.m.: Make My Day Juice

6:00 p.m.: Electrolyte Power Juice

8:30 p.m.: Electrolyte Power Juice

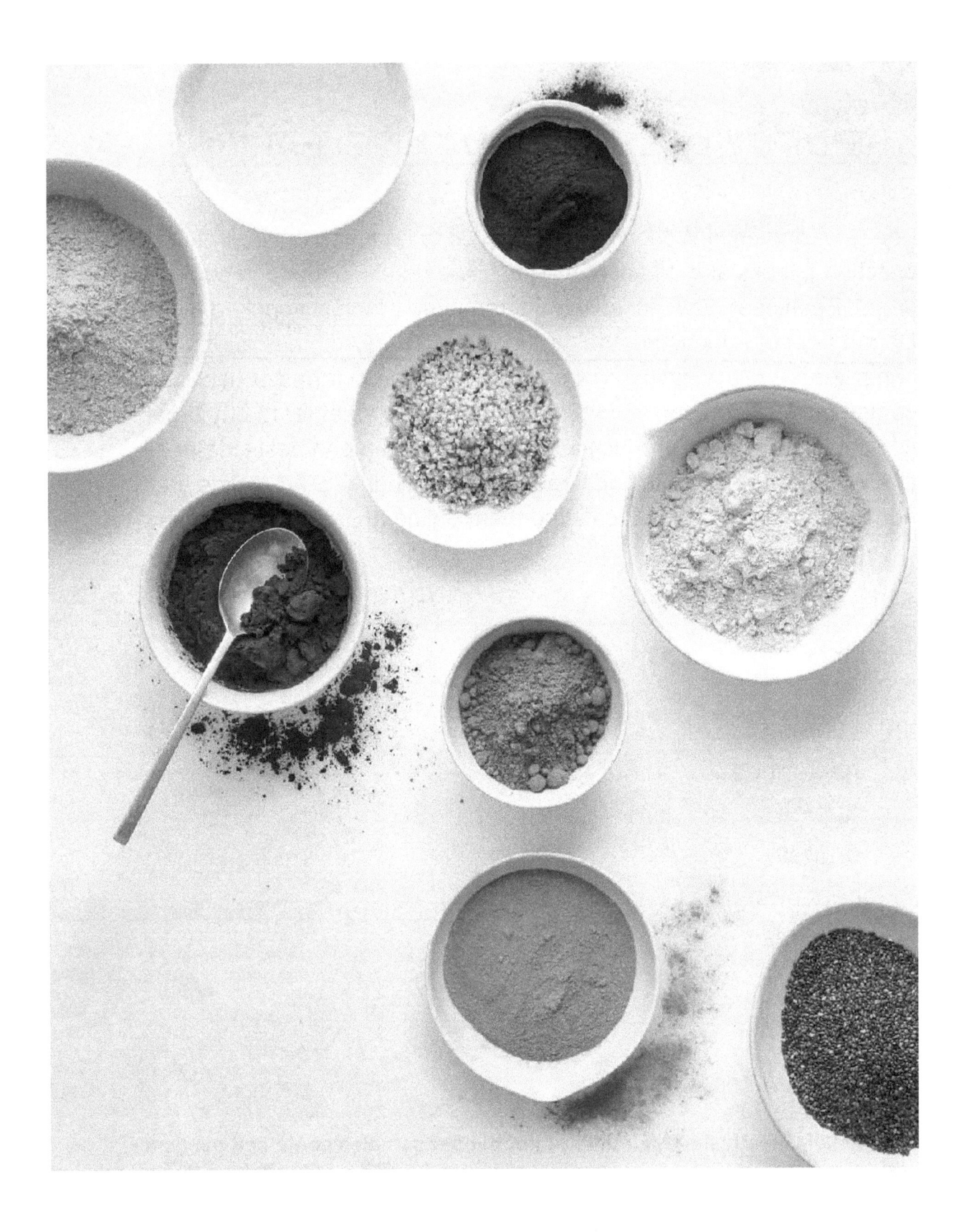

THE DIRTY DOZEN™ AND THE CLEAN FIFTEEN™

The Environmental Working Group (EWG), a nonprofit environmental watchdog, looks at data about the pesticide residues found in commercial crops. Each year, EWG uses that information, which is supplied by the US Department of Agriculture and the Food and Drug Administration, to compile a list of the dirtiest and cleanest produce in terms of pesticide contamination. You can use these lists to decide whether to buy organic or conventionally grown produce. Organic does not mean pesticide-free, though, so wash all fruits and vegetables thoroughly. EWG's lists are updated annually, and you can find them online at EWG.org/FoodNews.

Dirty Dozen™

1. strawberries
2. spinach
3. kale
4. nectarines
5. apples
6. grapes
7. peaches
8. cherries
9. pears
10. tomatoes
11. celery
12. potatoes

Additionally, nearly three-quarters of hot pepper samples contained pesticide residues.

Clean Fifteen™

1. avocados
2. sweet corn
3. pineapples
4. sweet peas (frozen)
5. onions
6. papayas
7. eggplants
8. asparagus
9. kiwis
10. cabbages
11. cauliflower
12. cantaloupes
13. broccoli
14. mushrooms
15. honeydew melons

MEASUREMENT CONVERSIONS

VOLUME EQUIVALENTS (LIQUID)

US STANDARD	US STANDARD (OUNCES)	METRIC (APPROXIMATE)
2 tablespoons	1 fl. oz.	30 mL
¼ cup	2 fl. oz.	60 mL
½ cup	4 fl. oz.	120 mL
1 cup	8 fl. oz.	240 mL
1½ cups	12 fl. oz.	355 mL
2 cups or 1 pint	16 fl. oz.	475 mL
4 cups or 1 quart	32 fl. oz.	1 L
1 gallon	128 fl. oz.	4 L

OVEN TEMPERATURES

FAHRENHEIT (F)	CELSIUS (C) (APPROXIMATE)
250°F	120°C
300°F	150°C
325°F	165°C
350°F	180°C
375°F	190°C
400°F	200°C
425°F	220°C
450°F	230°C

VOLUME EQUIVALENTS (DRY)

US STANDARD	METRIC (APPROXIMATE)
⅛ teaspoon	0.5 mL
¼ teaspoon	1 mL
½ teaspoon	2 mL
¾ teaspoon	4 mL
1 teaspoon	5 mL
1 tablespoon	15 mL
¼ cup	59 mL
⅓ cup	79 mL
½ cup	118 mL
⅔ cup	156 mL
¾ cup	177 mL
1 cup	235 mL
2 cups or 1 pint	475 mL
3 cups	700 mL
4 cups or 1 quart	1 L

WEIGHT EQUIVALENTS

US STANDARD	METRIC (APPROXIMATE)
½ ounce	15 g
1 ounce	30 g
2 ounces	60 g
4 ounces	115 g
8 ounces	225 g
12 ounces	340 g
16 ounces or 1 pound	455 g

CPSIA information can be obtained
at www.ICGtesting.com
Printed in the USA
BVHW061442220621
610213BV00002B/417